# THE NURSING AUDIT
## self-regulation in nursing practice

### Second Edition

# THE NURSING AUDIT

## self-regulation in nursing practice

## Second Edition

**Maria C. Phaneuf, R.N., M.A.**

*Professor Emeritus*
*College of Nursing*
*Wayne State University*
*Detroit, Michigan*

APPLETON-CENTURY-CROFTS/New York

**Library of Congress Cataloging in Publication Data**

Phaneuf, Maria C
   The nursing audit.

   Includes index.
   1. Nursing audit. [DNLM: 1. Nursing audit.
WY100 P535n]
RT85.5.P48  1976      658.5'62     76-21719
ISBN 0-8385-7005-4

Copyright © 1976 by APPLETON-CENTURY-CROFTS
A Publishing Division of Prentice-Hall, Inc.

76 77 78 79 80 / 10 9 8 7 6 5 4 3 2 1

Prentice-Hall International, Inc., London
Prentice-Hall of Australia, Pty. Ltd., Sydney
Prentice-Hall of India Private Limited, New Delhi
Prentice-Hall of Japan, Inc., Tokyo
Prentice-Hall of Southeast Asia (Pte.) Ltd., Singapore

Printed in the United States of America

*To nurses and the people who depend on them*

# CONTRIBUTORS

**Ruth J. Husung, R.N., M.A.**

Coordinator, Departmental Relations
Department of Nursing
University of Michigan Hospital
Ann Arbor, Michigan

**Norma M. Lang, R.N., Ph.D.**

Associate Professor
University of Wisconsin-Milwaukee,
School of Nursing
Milwaukee, Wisconsin

**Sylvia R. Peabody, R.N., M.Sc.**

Executive Director,
Visiting Nurse Agency of Metropolitan Detroit
Detroit, Michigan

**Maria C. Phaneuf, R.N., M.A.**

Professor Emeritus
College of Nursing
Wayne State University
Detroit, Michigan

**Mabel A. Wandelt, R.N., Ph.D.**

Acting Dean,
College of Nursing
University of Delaware
Newark, Delaware

**Marie J. Zimmer, R.N., M.S.N., F.A.A.N.**

Director of Nursing Service and Clinical Professor,
School of Nursing,
University of Wisconsin,
Madison, Wisconsin

# PREFACE

The Nursing Audit: Self-regulation in Nursing Practice is the second edition of The Nursing Audit: Profile for Excellence. As the title connotes, the second edition reflects advancement of nursing as a human service profession; because of the progress, perspectives directed to further advancement are now offered. At the same time, the book remains a guide for nursing administrators and staffs who wish regularly to use the originally delineated audit as one method of quality control in hospitals, nursing facilities, public health nursing agencies, ambulatory care centers, and any other settings in which nursing is a basic service.

Other people involved in community health services, education for the health professions, continuing education in nursing, and research pertinent to service and education, who are concerned with the quality of care may find some uses for the new edition.

This book offers the following contributions:

1. It asserts nursing responsibility and authority for nursing measurement and control of the quality of nursing care as a moral obligation.
2. It delineates systematic use of the patient-centered nursing audit to answer the question, "What is the quality of care provided?" The answer to the question entails nurses' use of criterion measures based on the seven functions of nursing to develop quantified data from which baseline and subsequent quality profiles can be drawn.
3. It presents illustrations of the initiation and continued use of the audit in hospitals, nursing homes, and public health agencies, along with improvement in the quality of care that results from strategic use of audit findings.
4. It provides an excerpt from a table of random numbers with directions for use in selecting valid samples of patient care records for auditing, as well as audit forms that include permission to reproduce them.
5. Contributed chapters provide special offerings.
6. It offers concepts and conceptualizations germane to nursing and to health service systems that can be useful in intensifying nursing involvement at all levels for the improvement of the care and the health of people whose lives are or could be influenced through professional nursing practice.

My indebtedness to individuals and organizations as expressed in the preface of the first edition continues over time. The circle of indebtedness has enlarged.

Ruth Husung, Norma Lang, Sylvia Peabody, Mabel Wandelt, and Marie Zimmer, are due special thanks not only for their contributions that enrich the second edition, but also for the privilege of association with them in other contexts.

Father Walter A. Markowicz has not only provided me with an example of an ethician in action; he has also reviewed and commented on parts of the book that relate to ethics and morality.

Beaufort Cranford reviewed sections of the book that were of particular interest to him, and made suggestions for improvement, most of which I have used.

Dorothy Reilly was a special source of encouragement; she clearly sees the parallels between the potentials and problems in quality appraisal of nursing service and the potentials and problems in quality appraisal in nursing education, including continuing education.

To the physicians, clinical pharmacists, and social workers who have assessed my efforts and contributed to my interdisciplinary knowledge and perspective, I am grateful.

My indebtedness to Avedis Donabedian is shown by the liberal use I have made of and the liberties I have taken with his ideas. Without the fruits of his scholarly endeavors, my work would have been seriously limited.

A profound debt is owed to the many nurses in the United States and Canada who used the earlier book, stimulated my thinking, and otherwise encouraged me by caring so much about patients and about nursing. Because of them, the second book is now offered.

*M.C. Phaneuf*
*October 15, 1975*

# CONTENTS

# Foreword to the First Edition

There is a "social contract" between society and the professions. Under its terms, society grants the professions authority over functions vital to itself and permits them considerable autonomy in the conduct of their own affairs. In return, the professions are expected to act responsibly, always mindful of the public trust. Self-regulation to assure quality in performance is at the heart of this relationship. It is the authentic hallmark of a mature profession.

In this respect, nursing has had a long, distinguished, almost enviable, tradition. No other profession has been more sensitive to its public obligations or more assiduous in self-examination. If anything, such self-examination has at times, been too harsh, too self-deprecating. It has, however, produced a body of literature on the quality of nursing care that is remarkable for the breadth of its concerns, the richness of its content, and the inventiveness of its methods. This volume by Maria Phaneuf will, no doubt, occupy an honored place in this distinguished company.

The subject of quality of nursing ordinarily brings to mind the general hospital. The nurses are envisaged organized in their tight hierarchies, many levels deep, each level watchful over the ranks beneath. In such a system, quality is presumed to be assured through direct and constant supervision. There appears to be less need for mechanisms of "peer review" that play such a prominent role in that other health profession—medicine! But nursing no longer fits this comfortable stereotype. Increasingly, the nurse is to be found in the extended care facility, the community agency, the neighborhood health center, and in the patient's home. At the same time, in every setting, the scope of her responsibilities and of her competence has expanded considerably. More and more, the nurse functions as an autonomous professional, equal to other members in a team, and subject only to remote and tenuous supervision by administrative superiors. Under these circumstances the nursing audit becomes an

essential tool through which the profession honors its "social contract." The audit recognizes, at the same time, the autonomy of the
individual practitioner and the collegiality of the profession. It also
declares, without equivocation, that only nurses are competent to
evaluate nursing care.

Many methods have been used to evaluate health care, in general, and nursing care, in particular. Some have concerned themselves with identifying those elements in the setting which are
thought to influence performance. Others have measured the outcomes of care defined as states of health or well-being. Still others
have examined the process of care itself in search for evidence that
bears on professional judgment and performance. The debate over
which of these approaches is the more appropriate is largely
academic. Surely, all are needed if one is to understand the many aspects of health care in a given situation and to take corrective or preventive action.

The nursing audit focuses on the process of care itself. It asks
whether nursing care, as provided in a specified setting, meets standards of excellence formulated by the profession. These standards are
seen as professional imperatives, unmodified by considerations of
feasibility or cost. Furthermore, in the grand fiduciary tradition of the
profession, they declare what is best for the individual patient and for
patients as a group.

Quite properly, the audit begins by specifying those functions
that collectively constitute "nursing." Only one of these (application
and execution of physician's legal orders) is "dependent," in part, on
the judgment and instructions of another health profession. In the
performance of an additional six functions, the nurse acts as an "independent" and co-equal practitioner. Further, the emphasis is not
on the technical performance of tasks (though these are an element to
be considered) but on professional judgment and professional skill in
the discharge of responsibilities for patient care.

To achieve specificity and precision, the basic seven functions of
nursing are further subdivided into 50 components, of which there
are 4 to 16 per function. For each of these components, the assessor of
care makes a judgment on a five-point scale ranging from "excellent"
to "unsafe." Scores are attached to each component accordingly. The
procedure specifies the scores to be attached and the manner in which
they are to be added to arrive at a subtotal for each function and a
grand total for nursing care as a whole.

Several features of this procedure are notable. First, the judgment concerning the quality of care rests squarely on professional

standards and professional opinion. The specification of functions, components of functions, scales, scores, and methods of aggregation merely defines the manner in which professional judgment is applied; it does not replace it. Second, inherent in the weighting system employed is a set of values as to which aspects of nursing care are more important than others. Those who disagree with these values could, presumably, adopt others. It is even conceivable that the functions could be redefined and their components modified. But the principle fundamental to the method would survive these changes. This does not mean that such modifications are to be undertaken lightly. There is great value to adhering meticulously to standardized definitions and a uniform procedure. In this way, one obtains a maximum of comparability among settings and over time. Such comparability is essential if one is to obtain a better understanding of the relationships between professional performance, on the one hand, and the properties of the organization or the outcomes of care, on the other.

A third important feature of the method is the emphasis on the "profile" of care. While the capacity to arrive at a single overall judgment on the quality of care is a desirable convenience, it is often less distorting and more useful to examine the quality of care with respect to each function or even each component. In this way one obtains a detailed view of the many intertwined strands that constitute the fabric of care. Action to improve care can, as a consequence, be more sharply focused on particular areas of weakness.

Finally, the care taken in developing the measuring instrument offers hope that the judgments arrived at will be both reproducible and valid. Validity in this instance rests, most immediately, on the degree of agreement within the profession on what constitutes good nursing. This in turn must rest, ultimately, on the demonstrated relationship between specified features of care and the outcomes of such care in terms of health and well-being. A pervasive problem in all methods of professional audit is the great variability in ratings among judges who have seemingly reviewed the same materials. It is hoped that the careful specification of procedure, which is such a salient feature of the nursing audit, will reduce such variability to an acceptable level. A further precaution, seldom emphasized by others, is the effort made in the nursing audit to orient and train the audit committee so that reproducible judgments can be obtained. Finally, because the audit judgments rest on information in the patient's record, the veracity and completeness of the record set limits on the validity of these judgments. This is clearly recognized by the author, who predicts that one desirable consequence of the audit will be improvements in recording.

Too often, evaluating the quality of care is seen merely as a technical problem in measurement. Professor Phaneuf knows better. She recognizes that the effective implementation of audits in nursing, as in any other profession, is an intricate problem in social management. Accordingly, she devotes a large portion of her book to matters such as the constitution, orientation, training, and operation of the audit committee and the manner in which it relates to the director of the nursing program. She also deals sensibly and forthrightly with the implications of the nursing audit for relationships between nurses and physicians. Needless to say, not many of her recommendations and views in this area are supported by hard research. They do, however, represent almost twenty years of carefully considered experience with the nursing audit. As such, they command both credence and respect.

Professor Phaneuf makes it very clear that the nursing audit is an instrument with many uses. It is an administrative tool for evaluation and control. It is an educational device for formal and informal use. It is a research instrument that can be used to measure the consequences of changes in organization on the process of care and of changes in care on health status. Though not primarily intended for this purpose, it can also be used as a guide in the provision of patient care. Not least among its effects are the clarification of the professional objectives and the sharpening of the analytic skills of the reviewers themselves.

In summary, the reader will find in this book a description of the technique of the nursing audit as well as instructions about its operational and social implementation. However, the book is emphatically not merely a manual of methods and techniques. It presents eloquently a view of what is good nursing in general, as well as a more detailed rationale for the specific features of the nursing audit. With rare courage, the author also includes findings of the nursing audit in several agencies and a description of the consequences of that knowledge. Once again, it becomes clear that professionals often fall short of the ideals that they profess and that the pursuit of quality requires constant self-examination. This is not to say that quality is simply a matter of professional virtue or sin. On the contrary, the whole point of the audit is that it should lead to an understanding of the complex interaction between organizational structure and professional performance. The result should be a better environment within which better professional performance can lead to better patient care.

Needless to say, there is more to patient care than nursing. Accordingly, the author hopes that the nursing audit will eventually be integrated into a more general audit of patient management that includes the contributions of all the healing professions. Even more important, there is more to quality than the implementation of professional standards. At the level of the client-therapist interaction, there could be more emphasis on the viewpoints and expectations of the client himself. At the community level, there is the problem of assuring access to care. The emphasis on providing the best for those who gain access to care should not stand in the way of making an acceptable level of care available to all.

To raise these points is not to detract from the professional commitment to excellence which is at the heart of the contract between society and the professions. This book pulls us compellingly to this central point. It sharpens our sensitivities to the full implications of quality performance in nursing. It places in our hands a powerful tool to help transform our ideals into reality. For these things we owe the author a debt of gratitude. And we wish her book Godspeed as it ventures forth into the light.

*Avedis Donabedian, M.D.*
*Ann Arbor*
*May, 1971*

# THE NURSING AUDIT

## self-regulation in nursing practice

## Second Edition

# INTRODUCTION

*Our problem is not to find better values but to be faithful to those we profess—to make them live in our institutions.*

*John W. Gardner*

Health care is a human interaction in which services available in an institution, agency, or other system are selected for and marshalled around the patient in accordance with his unique pathophysiologic and psychosocial needs and potentials by professionals who are morally, as well as legally, responsible for his specific care. Individualization of care, therefore, is a value to which most practitioners subscribe. Few practitioners are likely to be satisfied with the degree of individualization customarily achieved. Some practitioners are worried about movement toward less, rather than more, individualization.

Institutions, agencies, and other systems are organized and administered to deliver service to large numbers of people. They are further influenced toward volume operations by governmental and voluntary programs of payment for care that are likewise volume operations. Efficiency and economy are values sought through the large-scale operations; with the broad and increasing application of technology, more pressures toward routinized uniformity rather than individualization and personalization in the provision of care may result.

Individualization of care in the interest of patients and efficiency in the interest of economy are conflicting values. This conflict must be faced and resolved by deciding which value will clearly and overtly be given priority. It is reasonable, however, to suggest that health care in a democracy, like democracy itself, must be judged by the way in which it honors and serves the individual. On this basis, the challenge in health care is the provision of personalized care to large numbers of people, combined with an efficiency that maximizes use of resources without sacrificing quality of care.

1

One of the ways through which nursing can meet the challenge is through self-regulation in practice, including quality assurance, with use of the results not only for continuing improvement of nursing care but to influence the shape of the future in the whole of health care. The challenge will not be met successfully unless the values that underlie nursing action are made explicit. If to be professional is to make conscious use of self, then we must know, as we are known by, the values that guide our actions.

The values that have been mentioned illustrate the need for their explication. On this basis, some ethical and moral considerations will be briefly presented as a context for use in examination of self-regulation in nursing practice as well as in the continuing self-examination and study of the ethics incumbent upon each of us and upon our profession.

The development of the nursing audit was a specifically value-oriented action begun in 1952. It was based on the belief that nurses responsible for the provision of care were accountable for its quality and, given an audit method they could reliably and validly use for the purpose, were capable of passing judgment on the quality. In other words, peer review was valued. The nursing process was emerging as the nursing modality; the projected audit method should, therefore, facilitate knowledge about and application of the nursing process. Society recognized nursing as a profession by necessitating licensure for practice; the projected method should take this recognition into account.

Pressures for governmental payment mechanisms were mounting. Provisions of payment for care were known to lead to increased use of health care facilities. Increased use of facilities could result in impairment of the quality of care unless quality controls were established.

At the time, there were no nursing methods for measuring the quality of care. Unless nursing could document the quality of its service, it would be in a weak position with regard to leadership in shaping the foreseeable changes in health care. The need for the development and use of nursing instruments that would yield quantified data about the quality of nursing was urgent.

Structure, process, and outcome could equally provide a conceptual framework for method development. The magnitude of each dimension precluded the possibility of one method that could deal in depth with all three dimensions.

The decision to develop the process-oriented nursing audit was made because the nursing process was likely to become a constant in nursing practice; use of the process could and should be appraised independently by nurses; because of the independence, a process-oriented method could most quickly be devised and implemented; and time was truly of the essence. The audit was conceived as one method of quality control that would remain useful for an indefinite period of time.

The seven functions of professional nursing[1] were used as the framework for the audit in recognition of society's sanctions and expectations indicated in nurse practice acts, and in order to cut across all nursing specialities to the broad base of nursing practice.

The seven functions are as follows:

I.   Application and execution of physician's legal orders
II.  Observation of signs and symptoms and reactions
III. Supervision of the patient
IV.  Supervision of those participating in care (except the physician)
V.   Reporting and recording
VI.  Application and execution of nursing procedures and techniques
VII. Promotion of physical and emotional health by direction and teaching

In the audit, the standard by which nursing care in any setting is judged is the good or better execution of the seven functions of nursing in behalf of each patient. To execute these functions is, therefore, to use the nursing process. Criterion measures were developed to be applied in measuring the extent to which each of the functions was carried out, as reflected in patient care records. The audit was designed for retrospective evaluation of the quality of care provided for patients as documented in the patient care records and with a focus on the patient.

Retrospective evaluation permits a reflective examination of completed cycles of care and identification of achievements, trends, and problems for total or specific populations under care, by using randomized samples of patient care records. Baseline and subsequent quality profiles are numerically derived representations of the characteristics of the quality care that are measured through use of the audit. The profile of excellence reflects top level scores for the execution of each of the seven functions of professional nursing. When this level of practice is attained, the standard should be raised, perhaps by statistically sound upgrading in the scoring mechanism. The present scoring mechanism was built into the audit after some years of experimentation in the use of the various functions and critical components. The functions are likely to endure. The newer nurse practice acts simply make more explicit the responsibilities expressed and implied in the older practice acts; through the newer acts, society recognizes maturation in the nursing profession. More stringent critical components for the seven functions can be developed as practice becomes more mature, more intellectually disciplined.

In practice, the systematic movement toward self-regulation is illustrated by the progressive development of methods for appraising the quality of patient care while care is being given, as in the *Quality Patient Care Scale;* for appraisal of nursing competencies, as in the *Slater Nursing Competencies Rating Scale;* and in *Evaluation of Patient Health/Wellness Outcomes.*

The phased-in use of all four methods in any given setting as interrelated and interdependent parts of a nursing system of quality of assurance would permit attainment of the goal of the system, and would be an operational affirmation of the ethics of self-regulation in practice.

Today, quantity, quality, and costs of health care are social as well as professional issues. One of nursing's obligations is self-regulation in practice that results in quality care. Granted such exemplary self-regulation, nursing can lead in bringing about health-oriented organization of personal care services characterized by demonstrated quality, adequacy in quantity, and the lowest cost compatible with the quality and the quantity of health care. The ethics of self-regulation lies in the doing; the doing reveals the ethics.

### Reference

1. Lesnik MJ, Anderson BE: Nursing Practice and the Law. 2nd ed. Philadelphia, Lippincott 1955, pp 259–260

# Chapter 1
# QUALITY APPRAISAL IN NURSING: SOME ETHICAL AND MORAL CONSIDERATIONS

> There is a social contract between society and the professions. Under its terms, society grants the professions authority over functions vital to themselves and permits them considerable autonomy in the conduct of their own affairs. In return the professions are expected to act responsibly, always mindful of the public trust. Self-regulation is at the heart of that relationship. It is the authentic hallmark of the mature profession. [1]

Nursing appraisal of the quality of nursing care, by whatever methods, is the sine qua non in self-regulation. Because of this, it is proper to delineate an ethical and moral framework, which obviously applies to quality appraisals as well as to the larger whole of self-regulation.

Self-regulation entails ethical and moral obligations. As here used, an ethic means a value-derived principle of good or right conduct; ethics means a set of value-derived principles. In other words, ethics provides the philosophic base and justification for action.

In the consideration of ethics, it is essential to distinguish between knowledge and values. Knowledge means the picture man has built up of the world that is derived from the most rigorous interpretation he is capable of giving to the most objective sense data he can obtain. It represents man's view of the world as it is. [2] Value implies a usual preference for means, ends, and conditions of life often accompanied by strong feelings. It represents man's view of the world as he would prefer it to be. [3]

Moral means the concern of or with the judgment of goodness or badness of human action and character. To be moral is to behave in such a way as to profess one's ethics in words *and* action. To be moral excludes being moralistic, which means behavior characterized by strong advocacy of specific right conduct and condemnation of all other conduct in others.

Additionally, ethics means an academic discipline, a systematic set of propositions that constitute the intellectual instruments for the analysis of morality. Three essential theories of ethics pertinent to nursing in a special way are virtue, duty, and the common good.

The theory of virtue deals with the character of moral agents, such as attitudes, habits, affections, and motives. The theory of duty deals with the nature of action, its objectives, goals, intentions, consequences, conditions of freedom, and voluntariness. The theory of common good deals with the social institutions that make and are made by good men acting rightly.[4]

Carried further, ethics lead to an ethos, meaning the disposition, character, or attitude peculiar to a specific people, culture, or group that distinguishes it from other peoples or groups. The American Nurses' Association's Code for Nurses with Interpretative Statements[5] and national generic and specialty standards[6] reflect a nursing ethos.

The national establishment of the Code as well as the establishment of and work for the implementation of standards are examples of professional concern with virtue, duty, and the common good. For the practitioner, virtue, duty, and the common good are involved whenever ethics are involved, as in the care of every patient and in special situations such as those entailing informed patient or family consent to diagnostic, therapeutic, or research measures; behavior modification; passive euthanasia; and commissions or omissions in professional performance. As indicated by the Code, care requires of nursing a value set or system based on core belief in the intrinsic worth of every human being, undiminished, unimpaired, or unenhanced by extrinsic factors, such as economic situation, education, professional or social position, or life style.

Ethically, the provision of nursing service entails evaluation of the quality of nursing care rendered to patients as part of self-regulation of practice. Therefore, there must be a primary focus on the appraisal of quality through nursing methods developed and applied by nurses. It follows that such appraisals do not entail validation of the appraisals by other professionals or laymen, though the appraisals (methods and results) should be open to others, as appropriate to the broad goals of quality assurance.

Nursing's right of, and responsibility for, self-regulation is being violated whenever other quality assurance or utilization review efforts preclude, impede, or exclude the use of nursing methods. These efforts may be exerted from within or outside of nursing. In either case, nursing's accountability for care is then in moral jeopardy. The challenging of the right to use nursing methods to appraise nursing care is a challenge to the nursing autonomy necessary to the control of practice. This autonomy needs to be asserted now on many fronts and always on moral grounds. Quality appraisal is a moral ground; an intellectually disciplined and united nursing stand on this ground cannot reasonably or for long be successfully opposed as long as explicitly moral means are used for the explicitly moral end.

Recognition of necessary nursing autonomy by those who challenge it is essential if nursing is to contribute to the health of the American people and the effective operation of our health care institutions and systems in a manner consistent with nursing's potentials for the common good.

Nursing autonomy as necessary to the self-regulation of practice is not to be confused with exclusive self-determination.[7] Such self-determination is not only incompatible with nursing's social contract, but is also inconsistent with what is known about the influence exerted by social forces to produce change. Many would probably agree that society has not hitherto expected nursing to be autonomous at the essential levels, creative, and capable of producing a broad sector of top leadership or leadership at the practice level.[8] To seek professional autonomy, however, is consistent with the nurse's professional responsibility to honor the public trust and contributes to making nursing itself a clear and constructive social force.

The attainment of necessary nursing autonomy requires consistent work. Recognition of the right of and responsibility for nursing appraisal of the quality of nursing care and the parallel right to and responsibility for collaboration with other professionals and consumers in the development of overall quality assurance systems would be a giant step to attainment of this autonomy.

Total appraisals of the quality of patient care will not be possible until each profession participating in that care accounts for the quality of its own practice *and* collaborates in multidisciplinary evaluations. Nursing will not give a proper accounting until it habitually produces reliable and valid descriptive and quantified data about the quality of care it provides and draws justified conclusions from the data for all to see, and for nursing to use, in improving care and health care systems.

Until this essential nursing autonomy is recognized at least in quality assurance, it is self-delusion to think that in most settings true partnership or collaboraton is possible. What is needed is the nursing policy of the pursuit of détente in working with whoever challenges the autonomy—whether this be another profession, a social institution, or voluntary and governmental bodies. Women, because of their female role socialization may find it at first difficult to work for détente. Détente implies power on both sides that is recognized by both; a recognition and acceptance of separate spheres of activity and responsibility; reciprocal acceptance of the legitimate interests of both parties; and some mutuality of interest and commonality of goals that are recognized by both parties. It is a little acknowledged prerequisite to genuine collaboration.

The pursuit of détente for the achievement of necessary nursing autonomy in quality appraisal requires specific use of an ethical base in which virtue, duty, and the common good are served, and the goal of appraising and improving the quality of care that human beings receive is sought through moral means.

Public confidence in health care is at low ebb. Nursing can be the health profession that leads the way in earning a new, deeper, and well-founded public trust if it works ethically, morally, without fear or compromise of principle, and with high visibility in quality appraisal.

## References

1. Phaneuf MC: The Nursing Audit. Foreword by A. Donabedian. New York, Appleton, 1972
2. Gordon WE: Knowledge and value: Their distinction and relationship in changing social work practice. Social Work 10(3):32–39, July 1965
3. Pumphrey MW: The teaching of values and ethics in social work education. Social Work 10(3):32–39, July 1965
4. Tancredi ER (ed): Ethics of Health Care. Washington, DC, National Academy of Sciences Institute of Medicine, 1974, p 4, 5
5. American Nurses' Association: Code for Nurses with Interpretative Statements. Kansas City, Mo., American Nurses' Association, 1968
6. American Nurses' Association: Standard for Nursing Practice, 1973; Community Health Nursing Practice, 1973; Medical-Surgical Nursing Practice, 1974; Geriatric Nursing Practice, 1973; Maternal-Child Health Nursing Practice, 1973; Psychiatric-Mental Health Nursing Practice, 1973. Kansas City, Mo., American Nurses' Association
7. Brown EL: Nursing Reconsidered: a Study of Change, Part I. Philadelphia, Lippincott, 1970, pp 2–3
8. Brown EL: Nursing Reconsidered: a Study of Change, Part II. Philadelphia, Lippincott, 1971, p 494

# Chapter 2
# SELF-REGULATION IN NURSING: A CONTEXT, SOME POTENTIALS

Self-regulation in nursing practice is one manifestation of professional accountability in health care. Accountability means being responsible and answerable for use of resources in the provision of service with regard to quantity, quality, and costs. Quantity connotes availability of and access to care, so that the right patient is in the right place at the right time, receiving the services necessary to his well-being. Quality refers to the essential character of care considered in the context of merit. Costs refers to amounts paid or required in payment for care. Quantity, quality, and costs of care are reciprocals; this means they are interrelated, interdependent, and interacting forces in the health care system.

Currently, "health care system" is a euphemistic title, because the primary focus of the system is on the treatment of disease and illness in acute care, short-term hospital settings. White[1] states the dilemma:

> Sometimes I am convinced that the American public and medicine's contemporary spokesmen have the same views of health and illness that they have of automobiles and household gadgets. Health and illness, it is believed, can eventually be understood in terms of physical and engineering models, and by the same logic, deals essentially with closed systems amenable to deterministic reasoning and convergent thinking. Repairs, adjustments, and an occasional new part, together with regular maintenance will ensure a long and trouble-free existence.
>
> As a result, center stage has been preempted by the modern acute care hospital staffed with specialists and subspecialists and supported by expensive equipment admirably suited to diagnose and treat diseased organs and malfunctioning body systems, but nevertheless singularly ineffective in coping with the problems of individuals and improving the health status of populations.

The focus on disease and the stellar role of the hospital are particularly disturbing when it is realized that estimates of illnesses medically treated in one year in large populations of affluent countries show that 89.9 percent of the illnesses are treated on an ambulatory basis, 10 percent are treated in hospitals, and 0.1 percent are treated in university teaching hospitals.[2] Patterns of quality control are primarily addressed to hospital populations. Patterns of utilization review are primarily designed for control of the quantity and costs of institutional care. Perhaps what is even more serious is the fact that health professionals learn how to provide service through care of a small and unrepresentative fraction of the total population.[2] Thus the sickness care system is perpetuated, and all the while, concern with the great problems of the quantity and costs of hospital care will delay if not preclude the development of a health care system. In such a system, there would be at least as much concern for preventive care and health promotion for the many, as there is now for care needed by the few when disease occurs.

The modern acute care hospital staffed with specialists and subspecialists and supported by expensive equipment admirably suited to diagnose and treat disease has a concomitant, which is the depersonalizing of care. This depersonalization is a trend that has been accelerated by application of computer technology, through which the computer may come to be viewed as the master in care rather than, properly, the slave.

Depersonalization of care has come about insidiously as the number of people using hospital and other care facilities has increased. Even more disturbing is the fact that depersonalization of care may be judged acceptable and desirable:

> The computer will play an increasingly important role (in the delivery of health care). Problem-oriented records are already being developed to assist computer analyses. The clinical and historical features of patients' illnesses will be analyzed by computers and correlated with the stored memory of the patient's medical past. Appropriate laboratory and other ancillary data will then automatically be ordered and interpreted; diagnostic probabilities and therapeutic approaches will be developed. The role of the physician will be one of clarification, sorting out and application of those measures still requiring human contributions. Physicians will probably be required only at the centralized facilities; specially trained assistants will provide the data from the patient. . . while the new systems of health care may militate against the development of human bonds—which we call the doctor-patient relationship—they will offer more medical care to more people.[3]

The diminishing of personhood that is often associated with disease orientation is commented on by a physician:

So he (the patient) petitions me for help before the throne represented by my office desk and then, as he leaves, he lays a sacrifice of money on the altar attended by the vestal virgin who serves as my receptionist, and next he heads for your hospital.

Exit lutes and zithers, enter clashing cymbals, falling bed pans, air hammers and the raucous sounds of the hospital paging system.

First, he discovers that he'll have to wait his turn for a bed, which indicates there must be other more superior people ahead of him. When he at last arrives on the day we appoint for him, the chances are good that his reduction in size will be kicked off by a put-down from the parking attendant. Next he'll await the grace of the admitting clerk and then he'll be numbered and tagged like a piece of baggage. When we place a tag on a person's wrist—as no other commercial agency does—we say, in effect: "You are so common and ordinary that we are afraid we won't be able to tell you apart from all these others."

Next, he is required to sign a form absolving the hospital from any responsibility—an act which scarcely inspires his confidence. Then he is assigned to a room. Were he to go to any hotel in the country he could always command a private room with a private bath, but now that he's sick and in a hospital he is not that important. As though he were a college freshman, the administration assigns him a roommate or two—or three. And not healthy, clean, intelligent roommates, mind you, but sick, groaning, smelly, diseased roommates with infections that can be catching. Finally, he loses his clothing—the last symbol of his power and individuality—and dons the hospital uniform. And there isn't any more ego-deflating garment than the gown that ties—and splits—in the back.

Man, like other animals, measures his strength by the territory he can command, so our diminished patient will often try to salvage a meager two square feet of territory by placing a few personal items on the top of his bedside stand: The inside belongs to the nurses.[4]

One of the sharpest reminders that patients are people has come from the American Hospital Association (AHA) through its statement on a Patient's Bill of Rights.[5] The statement reflects their recognition of the dignity of the patient as a human being, and that overriding concern for the patient should characterize all hospital activities.

Although the statement centers on hospital patients, the principles enunciated apply wherever people are receiving health care. A 1974 AHA survey that included hospital response to the Bill of Rights showed that of the 5,912 hospitals reporting, 56.2 percent accepted the Bill of Rights in principle, no action taken; 13.0 percent posted the Bill in central locations; 12.7 percent made it available to employees; 8.6 percent made it available to patients; 7.7 percent indicated endorsement of the Bill by the Board of Trustees; and in 8.5 percent of the hospitals, a modified version of the Bill was adopted.[5]

The provision of personalized quality care to large numbers of people at a cost the economy can sustain presents a problem so great as to defy solution. What can be done is to attack the problem by successively dealing with its components, and so reduce the whole of the problem to an eventually manageable size.

Mounting costs of care have intensified public, professional, and political concern with the quality of the care that costs so much. The voluntary and governmental authorities responsible for distribution of health care dollars (all of which come from the public) are deeply concerned with the quantity and costs of care. As never before, there is the possibility or the reality of external controls over quantity and costs of care, with varying attention to quality. External controls mean controls exercised by other than the providers of care.

Professional Standards Review Organizations (PSROs) are mandated through the Social Security Amendments of 1972 (PL 92-603).[6] The amendment authorizes establishment of PSROs under which practicing physicians will assume certain responsibilities for reviewing the appropriateness and quality of services provided under Medicare, Medicaid, and maternal and child health programs. The PSROs will recognize and make use of effective utilization review committees.

The American Hospital Association's Quality Assurance Demonstration program was designed for use in hospitals, with a focus on medical (physician) care. The program includes local criteria development, description of actual practice, judgment in evaluations, corrective action, and reassessment.[7]

The Joint Commission on Accreditation of Hospitals has added to its Medical and Nursing Audit Requirements.[8] The American Osteopathic Association continues to reexamine and revise its accreditation requirements.

Federal Utilization Review Regulations, effective February 1, 1975, for all hospitals that are providers under Medicare and Medicaid, aim to make institutional review requirements consistent with the PSRO review system, to create a single utilization review system for both Medicare and Medicaid, and to implement requirements of PL 92-603 (Social Security amendments of 1972). The regulations also stipulate care evaluation studies that are retrospective, in-depth reviews of known or suspected problem areas in medical care to identify these areas and to lead to appropriate action programs to make the necessary changes.[9]

Control of the utilization of services to eliminate overutilization and thereby reduce payments for care is a long-term trend that was intensified when Medicare became effective on July 1, 1966. Utilization review means examination of data to make sure that any given patient requires service in a given facility or other setting at a given time. If the service is judged not required, payment for it through the responding insurance mechanism is not approved, or if payment has been made, it may be withdrawn. The common baseline for utilization review is the average length of hospital stay for a given diagnosis, as actuarially identified over time. The "average stay" may or may not be a clinically valid base because the average patient is as difficult to find as the average American. However, the appeal and the logic of the use of average stays as utilization parameters is obvious where payment of thousands or millions of claims for service reimbursement is involved. Utilization review is directed to control of the quantity of care provided and containment of costs of care. This control is in the public interest. What is unfortunate is the tendency to subsume quality review under utilization review or, what is even worse, to assume that utilization review in the long run satisfies quality control obligations. The answer to the question, "Does this patient need to be in this facility?" does not answer the question, "What is the quality of the care this patient is receiving?"

Utilization review and quality review are based on different values, and the values are in conflict. In the interests of efficiency, it is understandably tempting to try to evolve single methods that will satisfy two purposes at the same time. But because money–large sums of money–hangs in the balance in utilization review, there is little doubt that in the dual purpose methods the quantity-cost values will outweigh the quality values.

The values conflict shows in another serious way. If utilization review findings are that a given patient does not need the services of the facility in which he is located, and quality review shows that from that point of view he should remain, denial of payment for the service may, in fact, be denial of access to care for him.

In broad terms, efficient utilization review may create a problem by turning general hospitals into intensive care institutions. If more people use hospitals for shorter stays during which they receive the same service that would otherwise be spread over longer stays, the per diem costs of hospital care can escalate beyond economic tolerance. In this event, some hospitals may be forced to merge. It is even possible that some hospitals would be forced to close for financial reasons.

The legislation and the programs and efforts that have been cited are hospital oriented and medically oriented. It can reasonably be anticipated that ambulatory and other types of care, such as skilled nursing facilities and home health care, will sooner or later be brought under the same governmental or voluntary umbrellas of control. Unless wise leadership effectively intervenes, patterns now being set will be followed beyond inpatient hospital walls and broadly applied with the advent of National Health Insurance or National Health Service.

The National Health Planning and Resources Development Act of 1974 (PL 93-641)[10] represents movement toward a national health policy and must be taken into account in action related to the quantity, quality, and cost of health care.

The Act contains 10 priorities which are to be considered in formulating national health planning goals. The priorities can be grouped as follows[11]:

1. Primary care service should be available to those populations presently underserved.
2. Comprehensive "systems" should be developed to include all services. These should include sharing agreements between institutions and subsystems, the formation of group practices as parts of systems rather than as independent entities, and consolidation of high-cost, low-volume services and functions.
3. More physician assistants should be trained and used.
4. Quality should be improved.
5. Costs should be studied, compared, and, presumably at least, contained.
6. More emphasis should be given to disease prevention, particularly through better understanding of nutrition and environmental factors and by better education of consumers as to how to appropriately use available services and protect their health.

The context that has been presented is germane to self-regulation in nursing practice. It suggests that in order to proceed efficiently, it is necessary to understand patterns and trends, to identify issues, to identify the values inherent in the issues, to make informed decisions about courses of action that are consistent with nursing's professional obligations, and to act on these decisions. The context suggests the need to study pertinent literature outside the field of nursing, as well as that within nursing, for an in-depth view of the points that have been offered, as well as others that have been omitted.

No profession is in a better position than nursing to help in movement from a sickness-oriented system to a health care system. A brief description of health is necessary here:

> Health is the function of the individual in terms of his family, his work, his recreation, his position in society. Clearly, health and disease cannot be defined merely in terms of anatomical, physiological, or mental attributes. The real measure is the ability of an individual to function in a manner acceptable to himself and the group of which he is a part. [12]

It should be noted that according to this description, even a dying person can be healthy.

The health-oriented nature of nursing practice gives nursing an advantage that medicine does not have. Because of this difference, nursing clearly has a special responsibility to identify and to carry out its coordinate and complementary role relative to medicine and its role in practice, including the evaluation of practice that includes cooperative efforts, as well as self-regulation. The following delineation of the nature of nursing and of medical practice is helpful.

> In professional practice, the nurse's primary intellectual concern, and functions related thereto, is that of helping each person attain his highest possible level of general health. The practice focus is on assessing people's health status, assets, and deviations from health, and on helping sick people to regain health, and the well or near well to maintain or attain health through selective applications of nursing science and use of available nursing strategies.
>
> In professional practice, the physician's primary intellectual concern, and functions related thereto, is the diagnosis and treatment of illness. The practice focus is on differentially diagnosing and treating pathologies through selective application of medical science and the discriminating use of available medical strategies. [13]

Lest a hasty reader misconstrue what has been said as praise of nurses and a put-down of physicians, it must be emphasized that, in general, nurses and physicians alike care very much about what happens to the people under their care, and that for both professions, the goal for their patients is health. The delineations of the two practices underscore *primary*, not exclusive, intellectual concerns, each of which is so compelling and demanding that few human beings, if any, can successfully handle the double focus. Perhaps we should stop expecting that physicians do so. Certainly, nurses have problems and potentials enough in the development of nursing as an intellectual discipline to occupy their full efforts.

It is important, however, to recognize that in the appraisal of the quality of patient care through self-regulation, use of some methods designed in the context of nursing practice is required. Also, that in working with physicians in patient-care appraisal, the differences in practice approach should be clearly recognized and respected.

The focus on disease and the present pattern of emphasis on in-hospital populations in quality appraisal and utilization review is too narrow to encompass nursing concern for the health of people, in whatever setting. Therefore, nursing concern with quality appraisal requires extension through the use of some nursing methods that are applicable in any setting where nursing is a major component of service.

The depersonalization of care that characterizes much of our present health services is a challenge to nursing. Nurses are a part of the systems in which the depersonalizing of care occurs, and therefore, they share the responsibility for it. Implementation of the Patient's Bill of Rights is of paramount importance to nursing, and this is recognized in the American Nurses' Association generic and specialty standards that have previously been cited. In fact, these standards incorporate the Bill of Rights, expressed in provider-of-nursing language. On this moral ground alone, there is justification for implementation of the national standards.

Present legislation and programs that result in combined quality and utilization reviews require serious nursing attention leading to decontamination of quality reviews by utilization considerations. Nursing is probably the only profession that currently could provide reliable and valid descriptive and quantified data about quality that would help bring about this desirable result. If nursing can carry far enough forward with this, the time might come when quality reviews are so effective as to permit subsuming utilization review under quality review. In other words, a focus on cost-effectiveness, instead of cost-containment, is appropriate to nursing. If costs are contained through the provision of poor quality of care, whatever monies are spent are improperly used. If costs are contained through denial of access of patients to care, nursing has a moral responsibility to make clear that this is what is happening, and to set in motion the forces that could prevent it.

Self-regulation in nursing practice, like the practice itself, occurs in a broad social context in which there are complex dynamics, conflicting values, and finite resources. Self-regulation is a matter of conscience for the individual practitioner and for the profession. To satisfy this conscience, specific knowledge, skills, and methods are required. Nursing literature amply reflects recognition of the meaning of quantity, quality, and costs of care in relation to the health of the American people. The movement toward national health policy makes timely, and more strikingly important, nursing leadership in the field of quality assurance. Quality assurance in health services simply means to make certain that the care provided is of good quality. Quantity of care, however extensive, and costs of care, however contained, lose meaning unless the quality of care is professionally accounted for and found to meet or exceed standards. It is in this light that quality assurance as a basic part of self-regulation in nursing practice will be presented.

# References

1. White KL: Health and health care: personal and public issues. The 1974 Michael M. Davis Lecture. Chicago, The Center for Health Administration Studies, Graduate School of Business, The University of Chicago, 1974
2. Milio N: The Care of Health in Communities. New York, Macmillan, 1975, p 159
3. Ehrlick GE: Health challenges of the future. The Annals of the American Academy of Political and Social Science, July 1973, pp 72–73
4. Bates RC: The special needs of hospital patients. Read at Michigan Hospital Association Management Conference for Hospital Nursing Services, Bellaire, Michigan, September 1972
5. Special survey on selected hospital topics: hospitals' response to Patient's Bill of Rights. Item 2. Chicago, American Hospital Association, 1974
6. U.S. Department of Health, Education and Welfare: An important announcement to the health care community about the 1972 changes in medicare. Washington, D.C., Social Security Administration Bureau of Health Insurance, November 1972, p 17
7. Quality assurance program for medical care in hospitals. Chicago, American Hospital Association, 1973
8. The pep primer: performance evaluation procedure for auditing and improving patient care, 2nd ed. Chicago, Joint Commission on Accreditation of Hospitals, 1975
9. U.S. Department of Health, Education and Welfare. Department of Health, Education, and Welfare, Social Security Administration conditions of participation—hospitals and nursing facilities: utilization review. Federal Register, vol 39, no 231, part II, November 29, 1975, pp 41604-05
10. Public Law 93-641. National Health Planning and Resources Development Act, 93rd Congress, S 2994, January 4, 1975
11. Pickett G: Toward a national health policy—values in conflict. Paper presented at the meeting of the National Association of Regional Medical Programs, Atlanta, May 6, 1975
12. le Riche WH, Milner J: Epidemiology as Medical Ecology. Baltimore, Williams and Wilkins, 1971, p 82
13. Schlotfeldt RM: Planning for progress. Nurs Outlook 21(12):769, December 1973

# Chapter 3
# QUALITY OF NURSING CARE: A PERSPECTIVE ON EVALUATION

Three major approaches to evaluation of the quality of medical care, delineated by Donabedian, are the evaluation of the structure in which care is provided, the process of care, and the outcomes of care.[1] This brilliant formulation is broadly utilitarian; it is generally accepted as a basic framework in quality assurance, and the simplicity of the formulation is more apparent than real. Perhaps because of this, there has been out-of-context use of its components that has resulted in considerable polarization, particularly between those who extol "process" and those who maintain "outcome" all important. "Structure" has not had such devotees.

A more logical approach requires recognition that the structure, process, and outcome components should be encompassed within *systems* of quality assurance. In such systems, the interactive and interdependent components could be used to expedite the efficient achievement of quality assurance. Each of the components requires use of methods appropriate to it; that is, the methods used should have structure or process or outcome as their *primary* focus, in full understanding that each of the components influences the other two components. Each has its purpose, each has its context. Unless there is such reconciliation, more time, effort, and money will be lost because of undue emphasis on one or another of the parts without recognition of the whole that is greater than the sum of its parts—as the formulation indicates.

It may be that the polarization has come about not because the formulation was misconstrued, but because the problems of quality assurance are extremely complex. In reaction to the complexity and in response to related pressures for quality and cost containment in health care, perhaps it is human to seek, however vainly, the single, simple solution and because of this, to emphasize the purported value of one quality assurance component over the other two.

In any event, let it be clearly stated here that in proceeding to present further content and process and outcome methods, our concern is the ultimate attainment of the goal of quality assurance through a system within which the three major approaches to evaluation are appropriately used and orchestrated.

Evaluation of structure includes consideration of the purpose of the institution, agency, or program, and its legal authority to carry out the mission; organizational characteristics, including staffing patterns and decision making processes; fiscal resources and management; qualifications of health professionals and other workers; physical facilities and equipment; and status with regard to accreditation, certification, or other approval by appropriate governmental or voluntary bodies.

There sometimes seems to be confusion in the use of words that relate to structure, as shown by incorrect application. For the sake of clarity, therefore:

1. Accreditation is the process by which a designated agency or an organization evaluates and recognizes specific programs, institutions, or agencies as meeting certain predetermined qualifications or standards. To date, major accrediting bodies in service (and in education) have been voluntary rather than governmental in aegis. The Joint Commission on Accreditation of Hospitals is an example.
2. Certification is the process by which a governmental or nongovernmental body, as a unit or an association, grants recognition to an individual, institution, or agency that has met certain predetermined qualifications specified by the certifying body. The American Nurses' Association program for the certification of clinical specialists is an example of the certification of individuals. State certification of nursing homes and home health agencies to the Federal government as meeting qualifications that justify Federal payment for services provided under Medicare is an example of the certification of institutions and agencies.
3. Licensure is the process by which an agency of government grants permission to persons meeting predetermined qualifications to engage in a given occupation or profession and to use a specific title, or grants permission to institutions or agencies to perform specified functions. Licensure for professional practice is an example of the former; licensure of nursing homes is an example of the latter.
4. Registration is the process by which qualified individuals are listed on an official roster maintained by a governmental (or nongovernmental) agency. State registration of licensed nurses is an example.

All of these processes are ostensibly related in one way or another to the quality of services offered to the public. Current attention to quality assurance and utilization review suggests that none of the mechanisms have satisfied demands for effectiveness and efficiency in the provision of health care. All of the processes are subject to modification over time; people who are most concerned and knowledgeable about health care should share in decisions leading to on-going improvements. Nursing initiative with regard to modernizing nursing licensure laws is an example of such leadership. In medicine and nursing, the continuing education movement is in part the result of doubts about the impact of current licensure processes on continuing competence in professional practice, as well as concern for the self-development of professionals.

A positive relationship between good structural attributes of an institution or agency and good care is ordinarily assumed. For example, it is expected that patients will receive better care in an accredited facility than in an unaccredited one. Assumptions and expectations, however, are not acceptable as substitutes for evaluation of the care patients actually receive.

Evaluation of the process of care entails appraisal of all major and significant minor steps taken in the care of the patient, with attention to the nature of, the rationale for, and the sequence of the steps, and the degree to which they help the patient reach specified and attainable therapeutic goals.

In this type of appraisal, the national generic standards[2] set by the American Nurses' Association (ANA) should serve as the basis for judgments of quality. The specialty standards, which honor the generic standards, should be similarly used where clinical specialty nursing is involved.[3] It is understood that the provision of nursing care will entail the use of additional standards formulated by leaders in the profession; by leaders in large institutions, agencies for institutions, or agencies of similar size; or by leaders in a given community or a broader geographic area. But all of these standards should be demonstrably faithful to the ANA standards.

The problems of making professional judgments on the process of care are compounded by various notions about the nature of nursing. Use of the nursing process, however, is affirmed by the ANA standards and nursing literature as the dominant modality in nursing. Underlying the judgments of process, too, there are recognized and unrecognized assumptions that the process of care is directly related to general or specific outcomes of care for the patients.

Evaluation of the outcomes of care centers on the end results of care. Here, our problem is the definition of "outcome" or "end result." Shapiro suggests that "The term 'end result' refers to some measurable aspect of health status which is influenced by a particular element or array . . . of elements of medical care."[4]

According to Donabedian, outcomes are the ultimate validators of care; many factors other than care influence outcomes; outcomes may not be known for years; and they are sometimes irrelevant.[1]

Evaluation of the outcome of nursing care is made additionally difficult when nursing is viewed in a "medical care" frame of reference. It would be helpful if there were more rapid movement toward use of "health care" as the system identification. In a system so identified, medical care (physicians' services) and nursing care (nurses' services) become clear as basic elements. This clarification might make it easier to focus on the influence of those elements— individually and collectively—on the health status of patients.

In any event, a primary focus on the needs of patients rather than on the self-images of either discipline is essential to the definition and selection of potentially measurable outcomes of care. It is also essential to identification of the contributions of each discipline, as well as their joint contributions, to the end results.

Examples of health status outcomes are self-motivation of individuals to seek the highest attainable level of wellness; the making of informed and self-directed decisions about their own health, health care, and the health service systems that they use; acceptance of decisions that must be made for them; coping with illness and health-related crises; and the making of informed choices in the use of health-related resources.

Among the factors which complicate formulation of health status outcomes is the disease-oriented, hospital-oriented nature of the present health service systems. Absence, remission, and cure of disease are still used as prime indicators of health; broader definitions of health are not yet operational in most health service systems. The mobility of people and the episodic nature of disease-oriented care further add to the difficulties of using long-term outcomes of care for the purposes of evaluation.

In some situations, the irrelevance of outcomes makes it necessary to fall back on evaluation of the process. This is particularly so when death is the patient's final status, because with present knowledge, it is not possible to arrest the fatal course of his disease. In the event of death, the basic question is whether the process of care permitted the patient to die with dignity, in peace.

Three approaches to evaluating the quality of care have been outlined to give some indication of the problems of evaluation. Evaluations of structure, process, and outcomes are equally important. Pooled results of the three types of evaluation would permit a precise answer to the question, "What is the quality of care provided?"

The nursing audit is directed to evaluation of the process of nursing care. This approach was selected because it seemed most likely to lead to rapid development of one practical method for quality appraisal which centered on patients. Selection of the nursing process for study also had a purpose beyond the development of an audit method. That purpose was to help nursing movement away from concepts of care which are task- and activity-oriented, and procedure- and technique-centered. Such orientations result not only in the fragmentation of care but also in undue concentration upon the components of care with too little attention on the composite of care.

This statement does not deny or minimize professional obligations for knowledgeable performance of tasks with effectiveness and efficiency. Nor does it belittle the importance of carrying out procedures and techniques with skill. It simply conveys the idea that these components are means toward care for people and are not ends in themselves.

Nursing is blighted by task-oriented concepts. This is, in part, due to an apprenticeship heritage and to nursing's relatively recent emergence as an intellectual discipline. But it is also due to the fact that the same blight plagues the present systems of health services in which nursing is practiced. Thus, double jeopardy to the wholeness of care is ever present.

Health service systems are undergoing rapid change in the hope of accommodating massive demands for quality care, provided within the limits of economic feasibility. One characteristic change is the trend toward management studies of institutional and agency operations, which can be considered to have time-task orientations.[5] In hospitals, nurses usually comprise the largest work force, and nursing is a key service; hospital systems studies therefore devote much attention to nursing service operations.

These studies of nursing service reflect the task-time orientation—what is done, how long it takes to do it, for how many patients. For example, data are gathered to show how long it takes to take temperatures; to give enemas and bed baths; to catheterize patients; to do colostomy irrigations; to assist physicians in changing dressings; to give medications; to record the giving of "care."

Efforts to measure time-task relationships in health care are not only proper but also essential. In health care, time has a dollar value. Then, too, it is obviously easier to measure task performance in a time context than it is to measure, in the same context, the human interactions and transactions which are the fabric of patient-centered care.

However, for health service systems in general, and nursing in particular, time-task studies are not without hazards. Although numerical results can be used for planning purposes, recommendations based on them may be formulated as criterion measures of efficiency (equated with effectiveness?) in the mistaken belief that the sum of tasks and activities, and the performance of procedures and techniques, represents the whole of patient care.

Reports of management studies usually include forceful prose about the need to focus on quality of care, and about the community service purposes of the institutions, with admonitions not to use study results beyond appropriate limits. Yet, the fact remains that numbers in impressive array, followed by prescriptive formulae, usually outweigh prose when it comes to the logistics of a health service delivery system—the procurement, distribution, maintenance, and replacement of material and personnel necessary for planning and providing health care.

The gravity of the problem of task-oriented concepts of nursing for the public is underscored by some present methods of third party payment for health services of which nursing is either an organizationally conspicuous component or else the primary component.

The following example of Medicare regulations for posthospital extended care, with reference to "skilled nursing service," shows a focus on tasks, activities, procedures, and techniques. This focus is used to identify services as "skilled" or "unskilled." Evaluation of care is based on these identifications through application of principles and consideration of exceptions to the general rule which sharpen the focus. Payment for nursing care is contingent upon the evaluations; the tail of payment can then wag the dog of care.

SUBPART A—HOSPITAL INSURANCE BENEFITS. Sec. 405.126
Posthospital extended care; defined.
Posthospital extended care is that level of care provided after a period of intensive hospital care to a patient who continues to require skilled nursing services (as defined in Sec. 405.127) on a continuing basis (see Sec. 405.128) but who no longer requires the constant availability of medical services provided by a hospital.
Sec. 405.127 Posthospital extended care; skilled nursing services.
(a) DEFINED. A skilled nursing service is one which must be furnished by or under direct supervision of licensed nursing personnel to assure the safety of the patient and achieve the medically desired result. Skilled nursing includes:

(1)  Observation and assessment of the total needs of the patient;
(2)  Planning and management of a treatment plan; and
(3)  Rendering direct services to the patient.

(b)  SPECIFIC SERVICES: SERVICES WHICH ARE SKILLED. Based upon the general principles set forth in paragraph (a) of this section skilled nursing services include but are not limited to:

(1)  Intravenous or intramuscular injections and feeding;
(2)  Administration of oral medication where immediate change in dosage or medical procedures may be required because of undesirable side effects;
(3)  Levine tube and gastrostomy feedings;
(4)  Naso-pharyngeal aspiration;
(5)  Insertion or replacement of catheters;
(6)  Application of dressings involving prescription medications and aseptic techniques;
(7)  Treatment of extensive decubiti or other widespread skin disorder;
(8)  Heat treatments specifically ordered by a physician as part of active treatment and which require observation by skilled personnel to adequately evaluate the patient's progress;
(9)  Initial phases of a regimen involving administration of medical gases;
(10)  Restorative nursing procedures which are part of active treatment and require the presence of licensed nurses at the time of performance.

(c)  EVALUATION OF SERVICES AS SKILLED OR UNSKILLED. In evaluating whether services not enumerated in paragraph (b) of this section are skilled or unskilled nursing services, the following principles shall be applied:

(1)  The classification of a particular service as either skilled or unskilled is based on the technical or professional training required to effectively perform or supervise the service. For example, a patient, following instructions, can normally take a daily vitamin pill. Consequently, the act of giving the vitamin pill to the patient because he is too senile to take it himself would not be a skilled service. Similarly, State law may require that all institutional patients receive medication only from a licensed nurse.

This fact would not make administration of a medication a skilled nursing service if such medication can be prescribed for administration at home without the presence of a skilled nurse.

(2)  The importance of a particular service to an individual patient does not necessarily make it a skilled service. For example, a primary need of a nonambulatory patient may be frequent changes of position in order to avoid development of decubiti. Since changing of position can ordinarily be accomplished by unlicensed personnel, it would not be a skilled service.

(3)  The possibility of adverse effects from improper performance of an otherwise unskilled service does not make it a skilled service.

(4)  Skilled paramedical services involving specialized training outside the nursing curriculum are not skilled nursing services. For example, physical, occupational, and speech therapy are discrete

treatment modalities requiring specialized training for proper performance. A need for one of these therapies would not necessarily indicate a need for skilled nursing care.

(5) Any generally unskilled service could, because of special medical complications, require skilled performance, supervision, or observation. In such cases the complications and special services involved must be documented by physician orders and/or nursing notes. For example, the existence of a plaster cast on an extremity might require skilled personnel in order to properly observe for complications and adjust traction accordingly. Such procedures would be undertaken only on specific physician order and would be documented in nursing reports.

(d) SPECIFIC SERVICES; SUPPORTIVE OR UNSKILLED SERVICES. Supportive services which can be learned and performed by the average nonmedical person (and which are not skilled services in the absence of conditions specified in paragraph (c)(5) of this section) include but are not limited to:

(1) Administration of routine oral medications, eye drops, and ointments;
(2) General maintenance care of colostomy and ileostomy;
(3) Routine services in connection with indwelling bladder catheters;
(4) Changes of dressings in noninfected postoperative or chronic conditions;
(5) Prophylactic and palliative skin care, including bathing and application of creams, or treatment of minor skin problem;
(6) General methods of treating incontinence, including the use of diapers and rubber sheets;
(7) General maintenance care in connection with a plaster cast;
(8) Routine care in connection with braces and similar devices;
(9) Use of heat for palliative and comfort purposes;
(10) Administration of medical gases after initial phase of instituting the therapy;
(11) General supervision of exercises which have been taught to the patient;
(12) Assistance in dressing, eating, and going to the toilet.

SEC. 405.128 POSTHOSPITAL EXTENDED CARE; CONTINUING BASIS.
Skilled nursing services are required on a continuing basis (see Sec. 405.126) when the continuous presence of skilled nursing personnel is warranted. In determining whether the continuous presence of skilled nursing personnel is warranted, the following principles apply:

(a) FREQUENCY OF SERVICES. The frequency of skilled nursing services required, rather than their regularity, is the controlling factor in determining whether the continuous presence of skilled nursing personnel is warranted. For example, a patient may require intravenous injections on a regular basis every second day. If this is the only skilled service required, it would not necessitate the continuous presence of skilled nurses.

(b) OBSERVATION. Where observation is the principal continuous service provided, there must be imminent likelihood that

symptoms will occur that indicate immediate modification of treatment or institution of medical procedures. For example, pending stabilization of the condition, a patient suffering from arteriosclerotic heart disease may require continuous close observation by skilled nurses for signs of decompensation and loss of fluid balance in order to determine whether the digitalis dosage should be changed or other therapeutic measures should be taken.
(F. R. Doc. 69-12833; Filed, Oct. 27, 1969; 8:46 a.m.)[6]

These regulations—and similar ones that pertain to home health agencies—arise from outmoded stereotypes of nursing. The stereotypes prevail because some nurses, physicians, institutions, and agencies find them convenient for maintenance of the traditional status quo in health services delivery. Payment agencies did not create the stereotypes but do reinforce them through regulations and utilization reviews pertinent to payment. Payment is made primarily for the performance of tasks, not for a process of nursing directed to achievement of health goals by patients. Hence in auditing, the focus is on the nursing process. Thus, auditing helps intensify the forward thrust of modern nursing for the benefit of people receiving service.

Shetland makes clear the concept of modern nursing.

Nursing is essentially a process by which a nurse uses particular skills and knowledge to assist another individual, or a group of individuals, to identify and deal with health and sickness needs. The process is one of interaction; the nurse enters imaginatively and sensitively into the lives of the people she serves in order to understand their health needs, determine their perceptions of their needs, reconcile the differences between the two sets of perceptions, and institute appropriate measures in interaction with the recipient or recipients of her service. The content and context of the interaction are kaleidoscopic rather than static, changing constantly as one factor in the total situation changes. [7]

A model of the nursing process (Fig. 1) developed by Berggren and Zagornik provides a graphic illustration of care which is patient-oriented and puts tasks within the context of nursing intervention.[8] Tasks are only one element of the total nursing action.

The nursing process as described and illustrated is based upon, and requires execution of, the seven functions of nursing listed earlier. It follows that assessment of the degree to which the functions are executed yields appraisal of the process of nursing care.

The rationale for selecting nursing process as the evaluational approach to be used in the nursing audit has been outlined, but one point should be added. The nursing process is carried out by nurses and is under the control of nurses; this simplifies evaluation of its

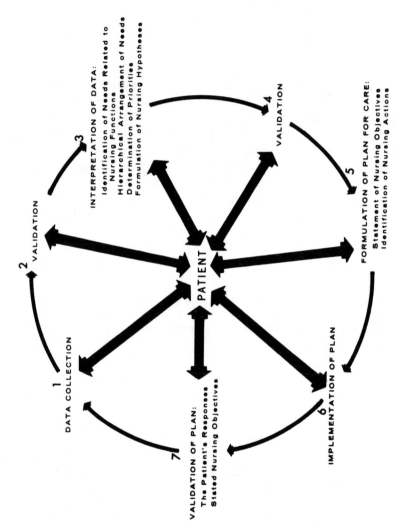

*FIG. 1.* Model of nursing process. (Courtesy of Helen J. Berggren and A. Dawn Zagornik.)

quality. The structures through which care is given and the outcomes of care are not similarly subject to nursing control. Because of this, the use of structure and of outcome as approaches to the evaluation of nursing care may be more complicated than the nursing process approach.

## References

1. Donabedian A: Medical care appraisal—quality and utilization. In Guide to Medical Care Administration, vol II. New York, American Public Health Association, 1969, pp 2–4
2. American Nurses' Asociation: Standards of nursing practice. Kansas City, Missouri, 1973
3. American Nurses' Association: Community health nursing practice, 1973; Generic nursing practice, 1973; Medical-surgical nursing practice, 1974; Maternal-child health nursing practice, 1973; Psychiatric-mental health nursing practice, 1973; Kansas City, Missouri
4. Shapiro S: End result measurements of the quality of care. Milbank Memorial Quarterly, Part I 45:7–30, 1967
5. Ludwig P: Establishing staffing criteria for evaluating nursing service functions—a management engineering contribution. In Is There a New Design for the Functions of Nursing Service? New York, National League for Nursing, 1970, pp 9–10
6. Proposed rule making section, 405.126. Federal Register, vol 34, no. 207, October 28, 1969
7. Shetland ML: Teaching and learning in nursing. Am J Nurs 65(9):12, 1965
8. Berggren HJ, Zagornik AD: Teaching nursing process to beginning students. Nurs Outlook 16:32–35, 1968

# Chapter 4
# WHAT THE AUDIT IS
# AND WHAT IT IS NOT

The nursing audit is a method for evaluating quality of care through appraisal of the nursing process as it is reflected in the patient care records for discharged patients. Patient care records include hospital and nursing home charts, public health agency case records, and other legal records of nursing service provided to specific patients.

Evaluation is a part of professional accountability. Nurses are answerable to themselves as practitioners; to patients and families; to physicians and others who participate in the care of patients; to the institutions and agencies in which they practice; to the community; and to the nursing profession which is in turn accountable to society. The audit is one way through which nurses can help to satisfy the accountability that is inherent in professional practice. It entails rigorous assessment of the nursing process actually used in patient care.

As previously indicated, the nursing process encompasses all major steps taken in the care of the patient, with attention to their nature, purpose, and rationale; their sequence; and the degree to which they assist the patient reach specific and attainable therapeutic and health goals.

The seven functions of professional nursing provide the foundation for the nursing process; the essential character of nursing is encompassed in these functions. The delineation of the functions, as developed by Lesnik and Anderson, is a particularly useful one because of its simplicity and directness.[1]

I.  Application and execution of physicians' legal orders
II. Observation of symptoms and reactions
III. Supervision of the patient
IV. Supervision of those participating in care (except physicians)

31

V. Reporting and recording
VI. Application and execution of nursing procedures and techniques
VII. Promotion of physical and emotional health by direction and teaching

The first of these functions, application and execution of physician's legal orders, is the one area of professional practice in which the nurse is dependent upon the physician, who in turn relies on the nurse for proper performance.

The other six nursing functions are independently exercised. As Lesnik and Anderson have pointed out, "The overwhelming number of functions and the majority of areas of control involve obligations of performance independent of medical orders."[1]

Since all seven functions of nursing underlie the nursing process, it seemed logical also to utilize them as the base for an audit designed to evaluate the accomplished process.

Key components for each of the functions are identified and stated as questions to be answered during the auditing of each patient care record. After scoring, the answers permit judgment as to whether the quality of care for each patient is excellent, good, incomplete, poor, or unsafe. Judgment is rendered both in relation to each separate function and in relation to their overall sum.

The audit is designed as a quality control instrument for use by nursing administrators, supervisors, and staff. "Proper application of professional control offers the greatest opportunity for employment of professional skills in creating and enforcing standards."[2]

In considering internal and external medical audits, Rourke has pointed out that, "The audit done by the outsider serves its best purpose only as a pump-priming mechanism for assisting the staff to take those difficult early steps down a road so difficult and so complicated.[3]

Underlying this concept, which applies equally to nursing audits, is recognition of professional responsibility for quality control. Also, there is recognition of the impracticability of using external quality audits to bring about planned change in the direction of higher standards of patient care in a way presently acceptable to professionals.

The notion of external quality audits conflicts with the principle of professional autonomy that implies values originating with and justified by the profession—which is to say, a literally autonomic system.

In the decade which had elapsed since Rourke's conceptualization of internal and external audits, however, official and public concern with quality of care has been intensified by rising costs of health services and dissatisfaction with delivery systems. The idea that health professionals are accountable mainly and almost solely to their professional peers is increasingly unpopular. And, in the final analysis, the status of a profession may be bestowed, modified, or taken away by society.

The nursing audit centers on professional standards with a view to clarifying them, increasing and demonstrating adherence to them, and progressive raising of the norms of care. The hope is that the aggregate of internal audits will serve these purposes. If internal audits are widely and systematically performed, there should be little need for external audits. The method under discussion, however, originated as an external audit and can be used as an external audit.

In any event, auditing should be done openly. That is, the auditing method used should be known to all concerned with quality care. Then results should be used to improve care. And the entire process should be carried out as one expression of nursing's accountability to itself and to the various publics affected by nursing.

When auditing is thus put into the broader professional context, a problem not previously mentioned emerges that is related to quality measurement. This problem is the tacit or implied hope that the audit will somehow immediately help lessen or resolve many of the various difficulties encountered in work toward effective and efficient nursing service. Because of this, it seems sensible to explain some of the limitations of the audit before getting on with further discussion of it.

*The audit is not designed for evaluation of care while care is being given.* Other instruments are needed for this purpose. One such instrument is the Quality Patient Care Scale (Qualpacs), "designed for use in any setting in which nurses interact with patients or intervene, directly or indirectly, to contribute to meeting a patient's nursing and health care needs."[4] The audit provides a retrospective view of the completed cycle of care.

*The audit is not designed for use in evaluation of nurse performance.* Among the instruments suited for this purpose is the Slater Nursing Competencies Rating Scale.[5] In the audit, the focus is not on the *nurse* but on the *patient* and his nursing care.

*The audit is not a "patient care" audit.* Appraisal of the total care of the patient would entail physician appraisal of physician care, nursing appraisal of the nursing care, a pooling of the appraisals, and quality judgments based on the pooled results—an integrated audit. If social workers, physical therapists, or other professionals were involved in the care, their appraisals would become a part of the pool. The nursing audit is limited to appraisal of the *nursing* care of the patient.

*The audit is not an error-detecting scheme.* It is not an underhanded or secret plan with punitive potentials. Monitoring with respect to policies, procedures, and techniques is an administrative and supervisory responsibility which the nursing staff shares while patients are under care, and it is here that errors should be prevented or corrected.

The nursing audit does reveal errors, and sometimes they are serious ones. Errors uncovered by nursing audit are analyzed as to their nature and significance, and as possible indicators of patterns or trends. The analysis is then used in instituting preventive measures. If the gravity of a given situation warrants it, however, the nurse responsible for the error should be identified and called to account by the nursing administration.

*Improvement of patient care recording, per se, is not a primary audit objective.* One assumption underlying the audit is that nurses will record what they perceive as important. Hence, audit efforts are directed toward sharpening the focus on the nursing process and its importance to patients.

In summary, nurse reviewers make the final judgments of the "extent to which nursing care has measured up to the characteristics that are specified."[6] The audit provides a framework for the reviewers, which facilitates these professional judgments of quality.

## References

1. Lesnik MJ, Anderson, BE: Nursing Practice and the Law, 2nd ed. Philadelphia, Lippincott, 1955, pp 247–93
2. Michigan Hospital Association. The University of Michigan Study of Hospitals and Medical Economics. Ann Arbor, The University of Michigan Press, 1961, pp 30–31
3. Rourke AJ: Insuring high standards of care. Paper presented at the Post-Graduate Course on Internal Medical Audit, Denver, University of Colorado, August 12, 1960
4. Wandelt MA, Ager JW: Quality Patient Care Scale. New York, Appleton, 1974
5. Wandelt MA, Stewart DS: Slater Nursing Competencies Rating Scale. New York, Appleton, 1975
6. Donabedian A: Some issues in evaluating the quality of nursing care. Am J Public Health 59:1833, 1969

# Chapter 5
# THE AUDIT INSTRUMENT

The audit instrument is set up in three sections.

Part I deals with patient and institution or agency identification and questions pertinent to institutional or agency policy and procedure.

Part II is the chart review schedule to be used in answering the questions listed under each nursing function category.

Part III shows the final quality score and the related judgment in remarks by the reviewer which bring to attention significant items pertinent to policy, procedures, and practices identified during case review.

## PART I. HOSPITAL AND NURSING HOME AUDIT; PUBLIC HEALTH NURSING AUDIT

The first part of the audit is the only one in which distinction is made between hospitals and nursing homes (care given in institutions) and public health agencies (care given in patients' homes, foster homes, or other places of residence).

It was necessary to set up different Part I's for institutional auditing and for public health agencies to accommodate differences between institutional care and care given outside of institutions. Each type of organization has characteristic policies that are legally or otherwise important. The questions to be answered under the appropriate Part I are those respectively considered significant for all patients in the institutions or in the public health agencies.

PART I.  HOSPITAL OR NURSING HOME AUDIT

*Data must be held in STRICT confidence and MUST NOT BE FILED with patient's record.*

## All Entries To Be Completed By Trained Clerk

1. Name of patient:     2. Sex   3. Age   4. Date admitted   5. Discharge date

  (LAST)       (FIRST)

6. Name of institution:    7. Floor   8. Medical supervision    Private   Ward   OPD/Clinic
                                                □       □        □

9. Complete diagnosis(es):


10. Admitted by referral from:    Physician on staff    M.D. not hospital affiliated    Clinic/OPD    11. Via emergency
                            □         □           □              □

12. Patient discharged to:    Self-care   Family care   PHN Agency   Other specify:   Died   Unknown
                         □       □        □         □    □

13. If patient died:    M.D. present    M.D. promptly notified    Family present    Family promptly notified    14. If patient Catholic:
                                          Last rites YES   NO
               □          □          □                    given:   □    □

15. All nursing entries signed by name and dated:   YES   NO    16. Nursing entries show whether made by professional, practical, student nurse, or other:   YES   NO
                              □   □                                         □   □

17. Patients' clothing, valuables, and other personal items were accounted for in accordance with policy:   YES   NO
                                               □   □

                                                    YES   NO

18. Operative and other patient or family consent forms completed as required by policy       —   —

19. A. Were there any accidents or other special incidents?       —   —
     B. If yes, chart indicates report was submitted to administration    —   —
     C. Or, report is part of chart       —   —

20. A. Kardex in use       —   —
     B. If yes, Kardex becomes part of permanent chart       —   —

21. Nursing care plan is recorded in the chart       —   —

22. A. Nursing admission entry shows assessment of patient's condition:
                                            physical    —   —
                                            emotional   —   —
     B. Nursing discharge entry shows assessment of patient's condition:
                                            physical    —   —
                                            emotional   —   —

PART I.  PUBLIC HEALTH NURSING AUDIT

*Data must be held in STRICT confidence and MUST NOT BE FILED with patient's record.*
-------------------------------------------------------------------------------------

All Entries To Be Completed By Trained Clerk
-------------------------------------------------------------------------------------

1.  Name of patient:                2. Sex  3. Age  4. Admission      5. Discharge
                                                       date              date
    (LAST)            (FIRST)

6.  Nursing agency:                 7.  Number of visits to patient by agency:

-------------------------------------------------------------------------------------

8.  Complete diagnosis(es):

-------------------------------------------------------------------------------------

9.  Was patient hospitalized immediately    10.  Medical supervision:
    prior to PHN service:                         Private    Ward   OPD/Clinic
    YES   No. days   NO   Unknown
    ☐       ☐        ☐      ☐                        ☐        ☐        ☐

-------------------------------------------------------------------------------------

11. Patient referred to PHN by:
    Hospital    Hospital                  Patient's   Other,
    Nurse       Social Worker   M.D.      Family      specify:              Unknown
    ☐           ☐               ☐         ☐           ☐                     ☐

-------------------------------------------------------------------------------------

12. Patient discharged from PHN to:
                Family                           Other PHN    Other,
    Self-care   care    Rehospitalized   Died    agency       specify:      Unknown
    ☐           ☐       ☐                ☐       ☐            ☐             ☐

-------------------------------------------------------------------------------------

13. All nursing entries signed by    14.  Nursing entries show whether made by public
    name and dated:                       health, professional, practical, student
       YES        NO                       nurse, physiotherapist, other:   YES    NO
       ☐          ☐                                                         ☐      ☐

-------------------------------------------------------------------------------------

15. Nursing care plan is recorded:        YES   NO
                                          ☐     ☐

-------------------------------------------------------------------------------------

                                                                         YES    NO
16. Were there any accidents or special incidents?
    A.  If yes, chart indicates report was submitted to administration    ___    ___
    B.  Or, report is part of the chart                                   ___    ___

17. Nursing admission entry shows assessment of patient's condition:
                                              physical                    ___    ___
                                              emotional                   ___    ___

18. Nursing discharge entry shows assessment of patient's condition:
                                              physical                    ___    ___
                                              emotional                   ___    ___
-------------------------------------------------------------------------------------

These answers are not scored. Where necessary, they are reflected in the remarks section in Part III of the completed audit.

Review of the two versions of Part I shows the differences between them; similarities are also obvious. It should be noted that Part I is set up for completion by trained clerks. Nursing judgment is not required for completion of these nonqualitative items; nursing time and effort in auditing ought not to be used where nursing judgment is not required.

# PART II. NURSING AUDIT CHART REVIEW SCHEDULE

The second part of the audit is the chart review schedule; the word "chart" is used to designate patient care records of whatever type. The schedule is used by nurse auditors who are carrying out the quality evaluation.

In the audit, the seven functions of nursing are used as objectives to be individually and collectively attained by nurses in the care of patients. The objectives are stated in terms of actions by nurses in relation to each patient.

Evaluation requires appraisal of the extent or degree to which stated objectives are attained. Evaluation entails measurement; measurement means one observation of a single phenomenon; and many measurements are necessary to formulate a generalized evaluation such as whether or not the care provided is good.

The degree to which objectives are attained is determined through use of criterion measures. According to Wandelt, a criterion measure is a "quality, attribute, or characteristic of a variable that may be measured to provide scores by which subjects or things of the same class may be compared with respect to the variable."[1] In this context, a variable is "a measurable component of an object or event that may fluctuate in quantity or quality, that may be different in quantity or quality from one individual object or event to another object or event of the same general class."[1]

The seven functions of nursing are considered to be the components of the nursing process, and, as such, they are subject to measurement. The components are complex, so it was judged useful to develop subcomponents for each of the functions which would serve as criterion measures for the larger component.

For example, application and execution of the physician's orders is a component that is basic to the nursing process and therefore to evaluation of the quality of the process. This component is more complex than it appears to be on the surface. In other words, the whole component has subcomponents, the measurements of which contribute to precision and speed in measuring the whole component. The measurement of the whole is derived from the sum of the measurements of its parts.

Basic subcomponents were therefore identified for this function. Each is viewed as crucial to execution of the function, and each is subject to unit measurement with relative ease. Each is a question to be answered by the nurse auditor.

1. Is medical diagnosis complete? That is, is the diagnosis(es) clear enough to permit intelligent execution of the nursing functions?
2. Are orders complete? That is, are orders clear, explicit, and inclusive when looked at in relation to the patient as well as to the diagnosis and other clinical data?
3. Are orders current? That is, are orders up to date in accordance with institutional or agency policy?
4. Are orders promptly executed? That is, does the chart show reasonable and appropriate timing between the giving of an order and compliance with it?
5. Is there evidence that the nurse understood cause and effect? That is, does the chart show that the nurse knew what she was doing and why?
6. Is there evidence that the nurse took the patient's health history into account? That is, does the chart show recognition that knowledge of pertinent points in the patient's past pattern of health and illness are vital to intelligent care in the present?

Key components were similarly developed for the other functions, with a resulting total of 50 subcomponents for the seven functions. The subcomponents range in number from four to sixteen per function. The focus was not on developing a standard number of subcomponents for each function, but on selecting those essential to the function.

Problems in the construction of quality measurement scales have been well delineated by Donabedian.[2] The reader in search of knowledge about the nature and scope of construction problems is referred to his work, because such delineation lies beyond the limits of an operational presentation of the nursing audit.

In the nursing audit, use of criterion measures was the first step toward developing measurement scales. After trial use of the functions and their subcomponents, without numerical values, technical assistance was obtained and the scale developed.

Large numbers of cases were involved and use of the instrument for even larger numbers was anticipated. The large number of cases and the need for seven separate nursing functions as criterion measures for each case resulted in the judgment that the functions' values should be weighted. Use of detailed subcomponents necessarily resulted in the development of subscores, the total of which would yield a final score for each case reviewed. The final step was to establish five numerical ranges in which the final score for each case might be ranked. A word judgment of quality was assigned to each of these ranges:

| | |
|---|---|
| Excellent | 161-200 |
| Good | 121-160 |
| Incomplete | 81-120 |
| Poor | 41-80 |
| Unsafe | 0-40 |

The following pattern emerged:

| Nursing Function | Number of Subcomponents | Total Point Value | Percentage of Points for Each Function |
|---|---|---|---|
| I. Application and execution of physician's legal orders | 6 | 42 | 21 |
| II. Observation of signs and symptoms and reactions | 6 | 40 | 20 |
| III. Supervision of the patient | 7 | 28 | 14 |
| IV. Supervision of those participating in care (except the physician) | 4 | 20 | 10 |
| V. Reporting and recording | 5 | 20 | 10 |
| VI. Application and execution of nursing procedures and techniques | 16 | 32 | 16 |
| VII. Promotion of physical and emotional health by direction and teaching | 6 | 18 | 9 |
| Totals | 50 | 200 | 100 |

Point values are assigned to the subcomponents within the total point value of the related function category. During chart review, each of the subcomponents is dealt with individually as though it stood alone—that is, as though it were the only question to be answered; and each answer is drawn from the chart as a whole. Definitions for each of the subcomponents will be considered in Chapter 7.

There are three response options for subcomponents 1 through 28. These items apply to the care of all patients. "Yes" denotes adequate evidence to support an affirmative response. "No" means inadequate evidence or absence of evidence. And "Uncertain" means that there is *some* evidence *toward the affirmative*.

Some of the subcomponents 29 through 50 may not apply in all cases reviewed. Here a "Does not apply" option is added to the Yes, No, and Uncertain choices.

It will be noted that the point values of subcomponents given to the responses are identical in pattern within each function category except for function II, observation of symptoms and reactions. Here, item 12, observation of symptoms and reactions pertinent to the patient's view of the course of his disease(s), shows a point value of 5 for an affirmative appraisal and a value of 2 for an uncertain response. Although there are two other items directly pertinent to the course of the disease, that is, item 8, observations related to the course of the above disease(s) in the patient, and item 11, observation of the patient's reactions to his condition, experience showed that the patient's reactions to the course of his disease was an identifiable dimension to which a point value should still be attached, though a slightly lower value seemed reasonable.

In examination of the subcomponents, it should be kept in mind that the measurement scale was developed after the subcomponents had been identified. In other words, the scale was adapted to the subcomponents and not vice-versa.

In summary, the general standard used in the audit is good or better execution of the seven functions of nursing; that is, the good or better carrying out of the nursing process viewed in this functional framework. The functions are specific standards that serve as criteria in the making of judgments. The criterion measures are the components that have been found minimum and essential to the execution of each function.

# SCORING: PART II. NURSING AUDIT CHART REVIEW SCHEDULE

After the examiner has checked the box of choice for every one of the 50 items, the total for each of the function categories is computed and entered on the Total Score line of the schedule. The categorical totals are added to yield the total score for the seven categories. The Does not apply columns are added separately and are *not* included in these categorical totals.

## PART II.  NURSING AUDIT CHART REVIEW SCHEDULE

### All Entries To Be Completed By A Member Of the Nursing Audit Committee

*(Please check in box of choice; DO NOT obscure number in box.)*

Name of patient: _____

(LAST)                                    (FIRST)

| I. APPLICATION AND EXECUTION OF PHYSICIAN'S LEGAL ORDERS | YES | NO | UNCERTAIN | TOTALS |
|---|---|---|---|---|
| 1. Medical diagnosis complete | 7 | 0 | 3 | |
| 2. Orders complete | 7 | 0 | 3 | |
| 3. Orders current | 7 | 0 | 3 | |
| 4. Orders promptly executed | 7 | 0 | 3 | |
| 5. Evidence that nurse understood cause and effect | 7 | 0 | 3 | |
| 6. Evidence that nurse took health history into account | 7 | 0 | 3 | |
| (42) TOTALS | | 0 | | |

| II. OBSERVATION OF SYMPTOMS AND REACTIONS | YES | NO | UNCERTAIN | TOTALS |
|---|---|---|---|---|
| 7. Related to course of above disease(s) in general | 7 | 0 | 3 | |
| 8. Related to course of above disease(s) in patient | 7 | 0 | 3 | |
| 9. Related to complications due to therapy (each medication and each procedure) | 7 | 0 | 3 | |
| 10. Vital signs | 7 | 0 | 3 | |
| 11. Patient to his condition | 7 | 0 | 3 | |
| 12. Patient to his course of disease(s) | 5 | 0 | 2 | |
| (40) TOTALS | | 0 | | |

| III. SUPERVISION OF THE PATIENT | YES | NO | UNCERTAIN | TOTALS |
|---|---|---|---|---|
| 13. Evidence that initial nursing diagnosis was made | 4 | 0 | 1 | |
| 14. Safety of patient | 4 | 0 | 1 | |
| 15. Security of patient | 4 | 0 | 1 | |
| 16. Adaptation (support of patient in reaction to condition and care) | 4 | 0 | 1 | |
| 17. Continuing assessment of patient's condition and capacity | 4 | 0 | 1 | |
| 18. Nursing plans changed in accordance with assessment | 4 | 0 | 1 | |
| 19. Interaction with family and with others considered | 4 | 0 | 1 | |
| (28) TOTALS | | 0 | | |

| IV. SUPERVISION OF THOSE PARTICIPATING IN CARE (EXCEPT THE PHYSICIAN) | YES | NO | UNCERTAIN | TOTALS |
|---|---|---|---|---|
| 20. Care taught to patient, family, or others, nursing personnel | 5 | 0 | 2 | |
| 21. Physical, emotional, mental capacity to learn considered | 5 | 0 | 2 | |
| 22. Continuity of supervision to those taught | 5 | 0 | 2 | |
| 23. Support of those giving care | 5 | 0 | 2 | |
| (20) TOTALS | | 0 | | |

| V. REPORTING AND RECORDING | YES | NO | UNCERTAIN | TOTALS |
|---|---|---|---|---|
| 24. Facts on which further care depended were recorded | 4 | 0 | 1 | |
| 25. Essential facts reported to physician | 4 | 0 | 1 | |
| 26. Reporting of facts included evaluation thereof | 4 | 0 | 1 | |
| 27. Patient or family alerted as to what to report to physician | 4 | 0 | 1 | |
| 28. Record permitted continuity of intramural and extramural care | 4 | 0 | 1 | |
| (20) TOTALS | | 0 | | |

PART II. NURSING AUDIT CHART REVIEW SCHEDULE (cont.)

| | YES | NO | UNCERTAIN | TOTALS | DOES NOT APPLY |
|---|---|---|---|---|---|
| VI. APPLICATION AND EXECUTION OF NURSING PROCEDURES AND TECHNIQUES | | | | | |
| 29. Administration and/or supervision of medications | 2 | 0 | 0.5 | | 2 |
| 30. Personal care (bathing, oral hygiene, skin, nail care, shampoo) | 2 | 0 | 0.5 | | 2 |
| 31. Nutrition (including special diets) | 2 | 0 | 0.5 | | 2 |
| 32. Fluid balance plus electrolytes | 2 | 0 | 0.5 | | 2 |
| 33. Elimination | 2 | 0 | 0.5 | | 2 |
| 34. Rest and sleep | 2 | 0 | 0.5 | | 2 |
| 35. Physical activity | 2 | 0 | 0.5 | | 2 |
| 36. Irrigations (including enemas) | 2 | 0 | 0.5 | | 2 |
| 37. Dressings and bandages | 2 | 0 | 0.5 | | 2 |
| 38. Formal exercise program | 2 | 0 | 0.5 | | 2 |
| 39. Rehabilitation (other than formal exercise) | 2 | 0 | 0.5 | | 2 |
| 40. Prevention of complications and infections | 2 | 0 | 0.5 | | 2 |
| 41. Recreation, diversion | 2 | 0 | 0.5 | | 2 |
| 42. Clinical procedures - urinalysis, B/P | 2 | 0 | 0.5 | | 2 |
| 43. Special treatments (e.g., care of tracheotomy, use of oxygen, colostomy or catheter care, etc.) | 2 | 0 | 0.5 | | 2 |
| 44. Procedures and techniques taught to patient | 2 | 0 | 0.5 | | 2 |
| (32) TOTALS | | 0 | | | |
| VII. PROMOTION OF PHYSICAL AND EMOTIONAL HEALTH BY DIRECTION AND TEACHING | | | | | |
| 45. Plans for medical emergency evident | 3 | 0 | 1 | | 3 |
| 46. Emotional support to patient | 3 | 0 | 1 | | 3 |
| 47. Emotional support to family | 3 | 0 | 1 | | 3 |
| 48. Teaching promotion and maintenance of health | 3 | 0 | 1 | | 3 |
| 49. Evaluation of need for additional resources (e.g., spiritual, social service, homemaker service, physical or occupational therapy) | 3 | 0 | 1 | | 3 |
| 50. Action taken in regard to needs identified | 3 | 0 | 1 | | 3 |
| (18) TOTALS | | 0 | | | |

TOTAL SCORE

FINAL SCORE

Example (hypothetical scores):

| Category | Total | Does Not Apply |
|---|---|---|
| I. Application and execution of physician's legal orders | 35 | — |
| II. Observation of signs and symptoms and reactions | 30 | — |
| III. Supervision of patient | 20 | — |
| IV. Supervision of those participating in care (except the physician) | 17 | — |
| V. Reporting and recording | 12 | — |
| VI. Application and execution of nursing procedures and techniques | 20 | 6 |
| VII. Promotion of physical and emotional health by direction and teaching | 12 | 4 |
| Total Score | 146 | 10 |

For computation of the final score, it is necessary to correct for the Does not apply items. Obviously, the final score should not be lowered by the value of items not judged relevant to the care of any given patient.

The final score is, therefore, the product of multiplication of the total score by the Does not apply value. The Does not apply value is selected from the following guide.

### "Does Not Apply" Values Guide

| Total of "Does Not Apply" Items | "Does Not Apply" Score Value |
|---|---|
| 0 | 1.00 |
| 2 | 1.01 |
| 3 or 4 | 1.02 |
| 5 or 6 | 1.03 |
| 7 or 8 | 1.04 |
| 9 or 10 | 1.05 |
| 11 or 12 | 1.06 |
| 13 or 14 | 1.07 |
| 15 | 1.08 |
| 16 or 17 | 1.09 |
| 18 or 19 | 1.10 |
| 20 | 1.11 |
| 21 or 22 | 1.12 |
| 23 | 1.13 |
| 24 or 25 | 1.14 |
| 26 | 1.15 |
| 27 or 28 | 1.16 |
| 29 | 1.17 |
| 30 or 31 | 1.18 |
| 32 | 1.19 |
| 33 or 34 | 1.20 |
| 35 | 1.21 |
| 36 | 1.22 |
| 37 or 38 | 1.23 |

## "Does Not Apply" Values Guide (continued)

| Total of "Does Not Apply" Items | "Does Not Apply" Score Value |
|---|---|
| 39 | 1.24 |
| 40 | 1.25 |
| 41 | 1.26 |
| 42 or 43 | 1.27 |
| 44 | 1.28 |
| 45 | 1.29 |
| 46 | 1.30 |
| 47 | 1.31 |
| 48 or 49 | 1.32 |
| 50 | 1.33 |

In the example given, the total score is 146, and the Does not apply total is 10. According to the guide, the value of the Does not apply total is 1.05. The final score for this case is, therefore, 153.3 (146 × 1.05). This final score fits into the 121 to 160 range on the grading scale, which is the good range of quality.

In considering the measurement scale, the purpose of the audit must be kept in mind. That purpose is, of course, to assess the quality of the nursing process through appraisal of the way in which the seven functions of nursing are executed in behalf of patients, with results that are subject to statistical analysis in the interests of nursing accountability and that can be used in systematic efforts to improve the quality of care.

# PART III. AUDIT RESULTS

In this section, the judgment of the overall quality of nursing care for the patient whose chart was reviewed is recorded as excellent, good, incomplete, poor, or unsafe; and the final score is shown. Because an occasional chart does not permit auditing, there is provision for indicating this judgment and the reason why it did not permit auditing.

The remarks part of this section is for use in bringing to attention salient points which, in the reviewer's judgment, warrant further consideration. These include: *specific comments pertinent to unusual nursing achievements* in the care of the patient; errors which require direct follow-up by nursing administration with the nurses involved in the error; items pertinent to institutional or agency policy, procedures, and practices that were ignored in the care of the patient or appear to cause unwarranted difficulty in patient care; areas in which clinical knowledge appears inadequate; areas in which the rights of

PART III. AUDIT RESULTS

All Entries To Be Completed By A Nursing Audit Committee Member
_____

Record reflects service as:

EXCELLENT (161-200)   GOOD (121-160)   INCOMPLETE (81-120)   POOR (41-80)   UNSAFE (0-40)

☐  (     )    ☐  (     )      ☐    (     )      ☐  (   )      ☐  (   )

Record did not permit appraisal   ☐        Why?


Remarks (including criticisms/questions pertinent to policy procedures, practices as
   shown in Parts I and II):


_____        _____

Signature of Nursing Audit Committee                   Date:
member who reviewed the record.

patients were ignored; areas in which there were problems in collaborating with others who participated in the care of patients; and any other matters that the reviewer sees as important.

# THE PATIENT CHART AS THE SOURCE OF INFORMATION IN AUDITING

The rationale for use of the patient's chart as the source of information in auditing is a simple one. The chart is a service instrument essential to the safety of the patient and the management of his care. It serves as the major means of communication between the various professionals involved in the care. It provides legal documentation of care provided. Recording on the chart is a part of one of the seven functions of nursing. The chart is easily available to authorized nurses for the purpose of auditing.

Use of the chart as a service instrument is inherent in the nursing process. In the nursing process model previously cited, the steps in the process are as follows:

1. Data collection, meaning the gathering of facts as pertinent to the patient and his particular situation. This includes direct observations, information about his previous experience with health and illness, and his patterns of daily living as well as other clinical data.
2. Validation of the data with the patient and others involved in his case.
3. Interpretation of data: identification of needs related to nursing functions, in the order which nursing care promotes, again with validation that also includes establishment of congruence with relevant theory.
4. Development of nursing care objectives and plans.
5. Implementation of the plan with the patient.
6. Validation of the plan with reference to the patient's responses and stated nursing objectives.
7. Repetition of the cycle as indicated at any step in the process.

Some nurses may prefer another way of formulating the nursing process, such as direct focus on problem solving, which is a systematic approach to the solution or alleviation of simple, complex, immediate, or long-term problems, characterized by an essentially sequential execution of the following observational, thought, and action processes:

1. Identification and definition of the elements composing the problem and interrelationship among the elements

2.  Specification of the crux of the problem, with consideration of the relevance of background facts and theories
3.  Determination and systematic collection of facts germane to the proposed crux of the problem
4.  Analysis, interpretation, and synthesis of the collected facts along with previously known facts and theories judged to be relevant to the problem
5.  Proposal of strategic courses of actions calculated to solve or alleviate the problem
6.  Evaluation of the proposed courses of action
7.  Selection of a course of action
8.  Action
9.  Observation and evaluation of outcomes of action followed, as warranted, by modifications of the course of action

Obviously, it would be impossible to carry on either of the described processes without using the patient's chart in the true navigational sense, as a map on which the course of the patient is plotted. And lesser processes do not yield patient-centered care.

Weed makes the case for the chart as a part of care. He speaks of the "medical record" and physicians; the concepts apply to the chart and to nurses.

"The medical record must serve the patient as well as physician, so it must be equally intelligible to all physicians, since patients are likely to require the services of many physicians and as much as possible progress of the patient among them must be easy and without confusion. The medical record must completely and honestly convey the many variables and complexities that surround every decision, thereby discouraging unreasonable demands upon the physician for supernatural understanding and superhuman competence; but at the same time it must faithfully represent events and decisions so that errors can be detected and proper corrective measures taken when lapses in thoroughness, disciplined thought, and reasonable follow-up occur."[3]

The concept of the recording of care as a part of the care is not, as yet, universally accepted. Use of the chart as the source of information is criticized on the grounds that it is the recording and not the care that is evaluated. The fact remains that, if recording is such as to preclude continuity of patient-centered care, then the care is in fact poor and may actually be hazardous for the patient. Continuity of care is an essential dimension of its quality.

Experience with the audit also strongly suggests that, as Donabedian says, "Good recording is likely to be associated with good care mainly because the conditions that bring about good care are also responsible for bringing about good recording."[2]

In a study of the quality of medical care in hospitals, Rosenfeld did show that there was a positive correlation between recording and the quality of care.[4] This study was one source of encouragement toward development of the nursing audit.

Use of the charts of discharged patients as the source of information was decided upon for several reasons. Retrospective auditing would permit appraisal of the completed cycle of service; final quality judgments cannot properly be made until the process of care has ended. The view of the process after discharge of the patient frees the auditors from responsibility for and possibilities of intervention in the care of that patient. This contributes to objectivity in appraisal because it helps to take the focus away from the nurse and what the nurse did or did not do, and to put the spotlight on the *patient, his* situation, and *his* care.

## References

1. Wandelt MA: Guide for the Beginning Researcher. New York, Appleton, 1970, p 314
2. Donabedian A: Guide to Medical Care Administration, vol. II, New York American Public Health Association, 1969, pp 14–96
3. Weed LL: Medical Records, Medical Education, and Patient Care. Cleveland, The Press of Case-Western Reserve University; distributed by Yearbook Medical Publishers, Inc., Chicago, 1969, p vii
4. Rosenfeld LS: Quality of medical care in hospitals. Am J Public Health 47:856-65, 1957

# Chapter 6
# PLANNING FOR AUDITING

The administrator of nursing service in an institution or agency is accountable for the quality of nursing care provided there. The administrator is therefore responsible for making the final decision that use of the audit shall be developed as a quality control operation.

Final decision should be made only after full exploration of the nature and purpose of the audit, with the nursing staff and with the supervisory and administrative nursing staff who will be directly or indirectly involved in or affected by auditing. At this time, other key people in the institution or agency who are concerned with quality of patient care should also be introduced to the rationale of the audit and to its method. Also, at this time, the means through which all staff and other key people will be regularly informed about audit results should be agreed upon.

Throughout the exploratory phase, and thereafter, there should be emphasis on the principle that nursing assessment of the quality of nursing care is a nursing responsibility in all settings in which nursing care is provided. The nursing audit is merely one constructive and feasible way of fulfilling a part of that responsibility.

When the decision to put the audit into operation has been made, the administrator then appoints the nurses who will comprise the audit committee. This committee serves as the professional nursing conscience of the agency through its monthly performance of audits, combined with its reporting of results and pertinent recommendations to the administrator.

The administrator should not be a regular member of the audit committee. Committee reports will be considered more objectively if the administrator has not participated in the process that yielded them. The administrator's use of results and recommendations is strengthened by noninvolvement in their production. In addition, the administrator as a regular member would inevitably influence the work of the committee, no matter how greatly he or she tried to shift away from his usual leadership role, and from the perceptions of it by others.

Requirements for committee membership include clinical competence and integrity recognized by peers; commitment to patient care and to nursing; interest in quality controls; and group work skills. The combined range of clinical competencies should be broad enough to encompass those considered characteristic of medical-surgical, maternity, pediatric, psychiatric, and public health nursing.

In general, one-year appointments for committee members are recommended; the year begins after the committee has completed orientation. During the final two months of the year, the committee should orient its successors.

Because of its goals and the qualifications of its members, the committee is prestigious. It also yields unusual opportunities for the professional self-development of its members, which can be realized in the course of meeting institutional and agency needs. For these reasons, the one-year term is recommended. This prevents long-term vesting of audit-power in one group, and provides for participation of as many qualified nurses as possible in the audit experience.

In a few settings, audit committee appointments have been used as therapy for "difficult" staff or other nurses, because the audit is patient centered, and audit committee service yields considerable professional excitement. In a few other settings, rotations have been too rapid for the good of the committee "to give the nurses exposure" to the audit. Appointments of this nature are not consistent with the previously mentioned requirements for committee membership. They damage the psychologic development of the committee, and its reputation.

Audit committees should reflect staff, head nurse, supervisory, and administrative representation. Additionally, the committee should include nurses not affiliated with the institution or agency that sets up the committee. A hospital committee should include a nurse from a public health agency and one from a nursing home. A nursing home committee should include a nurse from a hospital and one from a public health agency. A public health agency committee should include a nurse from a hospital and one from a nursing home.

Extension of the audit committee to accommodate nurses who practice outside of the respective institutions or agencies augments the pool of talent in the committee. Further, it helps unify nursing in pursuit of excellence, and fosters closer collaboration between institutions and agencies in the interests of patient care and community service. It also helps to minimize institutional and agency orientation, thereby sharpening the focus on patients and their care. For example, when, in auditing, questions are asked about a procedure in relation to a patient, the answer, "That's the way we do it here" might be acceptable within a given setting. Nurses not familiar with "the way we do it here" may be more apt to pursue the point in search of rationale.

In many patient care settings, practical nurses provide substantial amounts of patient care. Under these circumstances, practical nurses should be represented on the audit committee. The professional and the practical nurses should specifically remind themselves that there are four areas of practical nursing activity.

Environmental and physical management, and factual observation and reporting are the two independent areas of practical nursing functions. The execution of prescribed routine nursing procedures and techniques, and application and execution of legal orders of physicians and professional nurses are the two dependent areas of practical nurse functions. [1]

In some instances, the practical nurses chosen for committee service have not worked out well. Analysis of these situations suggests that either the particular practical nurses chosen were not effective practitioners, or that congenial relationships were prevented by a climate in which the registered nurse or licensed practical (or vocational) nurse ranks were respectively overvalued and undervalued. In any event, this problem is minimized or overcome if a registered nurse and a licensed practical nurse work together as buddies in auditing, and together they audit twice as many cases as would ordinarily be assigned to individual committee members.

An audit committee of no fewer than five nurses is recommended. In larger settings, larger committees may be required. Where small institutions and agencies are involved and discharges are few in number, a single joint audit committee could carry the audit responsibilities for a combination of an institution and an agency or for several small institutions of the same type.

A practical guide to committee size is that each committee member should review no more than 10 cases per month. A five-nurse committee could reasonably be expected to audit a total of 50 cases. After members have developed skill in using the method, a case audit can be completed in an average of 15 minutes for patients having hospital and nursing home stays, or periods of care by a public health agency, that were no longer than three months in duration. An additional time allocation of one to 1.5 hours should be made for an audit committee meeting in which the committee considers its findings, decides moot cases, and prepares the report and recommendations to be submitted to the nursing administrator.

The number of cases to be audited will be dependent on the number of cases discharged per month. If the number of discharges is fewer than 50, it is recommended that all be audited. If the number is greater than 50, auditing of a 10 percent randomized sample is advised. All the discharged cases should be numbered, if they are not already so identified, and 10 percent of them selected randomly, with use of a table of random numbers as the basis for selection (see Appendix 1). It is wasteful to audit more cases than necessary to yield a view of the quality of care provided in the institution or agency as a whole.

Review of all cases is recommended when the discharges are fewer than 50 in number because, in smaller patient care settings, quality controls in general are less specific or formal than they are in larger ones. As the quantity of care provided increases, formalizing of quality controls increases. In this sense, quality is in part a function of quantity.

There appears to be considerable distrust of sampling, particularly when the method of sampling yields small numbers of cases. There may also be undue reliance on large samples which may or may not be representative of the whole.

Instead of undertaking to allay distrust by theoretical explanations, it seems more useful to give an illustration of a practical approach to the problem. In one hospital, an average of 100 patients were discharged per month. There was anxiety about auditing 10 cases selected with use of the table of random numbers and generalizing about quality from the results. The anxiety was expressed by the director of nursing service and was shared by the hospital administrator. Because of this, 10 cases, properly selected by number from the table, were audited and results compiled. The 10 audited cases were replaced in the 100-case file, and 10 more cases were selected using other numbers from the table. This was repeated until six sets of 10 cases had been examined. Results were compared; findings in the six sets of audits showed a similarity which satisfied the administrator about the merit of the sampling technique. This exercise involved an investment of time, and therefore of money, but the cost was infinitesimal when compared to the monthly 100-case audit to which the leadership was earlier inclined.

Planning for institutionalization of the audit requires that arrangements be made for a quiet and comfortable room in which the audit committee can hold meetings, and for an area in which members can separately carry on their individual auditing at any time prior to the monthly meeting of the committee.

In institutions which have a medical records librarian, the librarian is a major resource. As a key staff member, the librarian will have earlier been introduced to the audit rationale and method. Procedures for the selection, use, protection, and return of charts should be developed with the librarian who must at all times know the location of any chart placed in his charge. The librarian should have a copy of the audit guide and related literature. He should be specifically apprised that nursing audit forms—open or completed—are *never* to be filed with charts, that *no entry* should be made on the chart which shows it was audited, and that there should be *no evidence* in the chart to reflect auditing.

The reason for this safeguard is obvious. Perfection in quality is rarely found in human services records; there usually are defects of major or minor importance. In a given case, evidence that the audit committee considered care less than sublime could be seriously misused if allegations of malpractice or negligence were to be made by the patient or on his behalf. In this event, the institution or agency which is making serious efforts in quality control would be unjustly penalized for performance of audits.

Clerical assistance for the audit committee is essential. A trained clerk who understands the importance and confidentiality of the audit can do all of the work on the audit that does not require nursing judgment. This includes preparation of the audit forms by completion of Part I; the completion of scores; the preparation of basic data for audit reports (summarizing data, such as age, sex, diagnosis, and other data from Part I). The work of the clerk includes preparation of data and translation of printouts where necessary, if audit data are processed by computer. The amount of clerical time required for work related to the audit is ordinarily less than one day per month.

Experience has shown that preprinted audit forms expedite the process and permit a variety of comparisons between institutions and agencies with regard to quality of nursing care. For this reason, forms that may be reproduced are included in this book.

The time to be used by nurses and clerks in auditing requires planning so that the work can be done during usual working hours, unless some individuals plan otherwise for themselves.

Using the guidelines that have been suggested, the administrator of nursing service can estimate the costs of institutionalizing the audit by determining the monetary value of the time of the various personnel involved in the auditing and adding the cost of materials used in the process. If a computer is used to calculate audit results, this cost should be included. The audit schedule was developed to permit computerization, but use of a computer is not essential.

One of the major areas which has not yet been touched on is the orientation of the audit committee to the task that lies before it and the development of skills needed for the method. This orientation requires considerable separate attention because the effectiveness and the efficiency with which the committee goes into and sustains action depends upon it.

## References

1. Lesnik MJ, Anderson BE: Nursing Practice and the Law, 2nd ed. Philadelphia, Lippincott, 1955, pp 282–87

# Chapter 7
# ORIENTATION OF THE AUDIT COMMITTEE

The main orientation goals of the committee are development of common philosophies of auditing and of patient care, and beginning skills in the use of the audit method. Work toward these goals is not so neatly divisible as the statement of goals perhaps implies. Work toward each of the goals pervades the entire orientation.

Development of a common philosophy of auditing requires excursions into the cognitive and affective domains of the individual members and of the committee as a whole.[1,2] At best, judgments of the quality of care entail intellectual efforts which recognize, and have respect for, value systems that influence those intellectual efforts.

At the cognitive level, the committee assesses and, if necessary, enhances knowledge of concepts, principles, and problems in quality measurements of care. In this context, the audit method is evaluated with regard to what it does and does not purport to accomplish.

In the affective domain, the committee obviously begins with willingness to participate in quality appraisal. Thereafter, it should move toward establishment of a generalized set of values on which the committee's work will, by common consent, be based.

The general course followed by the committee in developing a common auditing philosophy that has cognitive and affective roots is illustrated in discussions of "objectivity" and "subjectivity" which inevitably occur during orientation, and thereafter, in relation to judgments about the quality of patient care.

When asked to define "objectivity," committee members usually explain it as appraisal of observed phenomena that is uninfluenced by the emotions or values of an individual or group. "Subjectivity" is explained as denoting an appraisal, or proceeding from or occurring within an individual group that is subject to limited external verification. In other words, objectivity is a cognitive exercise the results of which can be replicated, granted the same observed phenomena; subjectivity is primarily a mental and emotional experience unique to the individual or group, with emphasis on the emotional components that obviously cannot be replicated.

The audit is based on the assumption that indisputable objectivity is not presently attainable in auditing—or in patient care either, for that matter. Human judgment underlies the questions and the answers in the audit, just as it controls professional provision of patient care.

The use of criterion measures in the audit, however, represents movement toward objectivity. In evaluating the quality of care against the measures, intellectual efforts are required, including those involved in analysis and synthesis, and validation of judgments either by congruence with pertinent theory or by consensus. Some subcomponents clearly connote belief in the uniqueness of the individual patient, his dignity, and his worth as a human being. Judgments with regard to these subcomponents are also subject to validation. The emphasis on validation increases objectivity.

The committee can evaluate progress toward a common philosophy by reflecting upon emerging individual and group attitudes and behaviors which stem from the philosophy. A few illustrations of desirable attributes may be helpful here.

A constructive attitude toward auditing becomes increasingly apparent. The purpose of auditing is to build, not to destroy. On the other hand, there is no place in auditing for fear or favor. Inquiries into quality should be as detached as possible. Findings should be honestly discussed and reported in a fashion that will encourage continuous strengthening of the nursing service and well-directed efforts to correct weaknesses.

Confidentiality about committee proceedings becomes a habit. Proceedings should not be discussed outside committee sessions with people who are not on the committee except in direct relation to committee minutes, reports, and recommendations.

A problem in auditing is created when committee members make chance remarks outside of committee meetings. A rift may then develop between an audit committee that says it is—and is in fact—operating constructively, and staff, supervisors, or administration who receive contrary impressions from the chance remarks of committee members.

The committee develops as a group in which members treat each other and the group with openness. Talents within the group are given full opportunity for expression and further development. Issues are identified and resolved, rather than skirted. The climate is pleasantly conducive to individual and group performance of appointed tasks; for an audit committee, life is earnest and life is real, but it should not be grim. The pursuit of excellence in auditing, as in patient care, should be gladly as well as forthrightly carried on.

Development of the common philosophy of patient care follows the same general pattern as that of the philosophy of auditing. To a marked degree, here also the philosophy of care is predicated on the philosophy that underlies the method. As has been indicated, this philosophy is one of belief in patient-centered nursing care, the process of which is developed around the health-illness problems of the patient who, in important ways, resembles other human beings but who is, beyond that, one special person for whom there is not a counterpart in the institution, in the agency, or even in the world.

Philosophically, it follows that the process of care is not in principle altered by the setting in which the patient receives care, whether that setting is a hospital, a nursing home, a public health agency, or any part of those establishments. The overall standard of care is that care be good or better, as judged by the separate and combined execution of the seven nursing functions upon which the nursing process is based. Default in the exercise of one of the functions faults the whole nursing care process.

If the committee, after thoughtful discussion, does not come to terms with this philosophy at least on a trial basis, auditing by the method under discussion is not likely to be fruitful. In that event, it would be better for the committee to resort to a method of audit that does not conflict with its philosophy of nursing care.

Skills in the use of the audit method are, of course, acquired only through thoughtful practice. The most important area for practice is Part II of the audit schedule, which the nurse auditor completes after a review of the chart. For this reason, attention is now directed to a detailed consideration of Part II of the audit instrument.

Each of its subcomponents is directly related to the function component under which it is listed. With this stipulation only, each of the 50 questions is answered as if the other 49 were nonexistent. Every question must be answered.

In the care of the patient, nurses had access to the whole chart for use in planning, providing, and evaluating nursing care. Therefore, in auditing, all data on the chart should be examined and taken into account—during the general reading which precedes auditing, during the specific reading needed to answer each individual question, and during the final general reading which is necessary to satisfy the auditor that the appraisal has been as fair as possible.

In assessing the way any given function has been executed, the auditor does not subsume under "nursing" those functions performed by other professionals, such as physicians, social workers, and physical therapists. What *is* of concern is the way the nurses follow up the care or teaching done by other professionals. For example, a nutritionist's note that the patient was given guidance in regard to a diabetic diet does not absolve the nurse from responsibility for finding out what the patient knows and understands about his diet and what he eats.

Even experienced auditors must *constantly refer to definitions of audit terms,* including those applicable to "Yes," "No," "Uncertain," and "Does not apply," as well as to definitions of the subcomponents.

As previously indicated, "Yes" denotes adequate evidence *in the chart* to justify the affirmative. "No" means that *in the chart* there is inadequate evidence, or an absence of evidence, to justify the affirmative. "Uncertain" means that *in the chart* there is *some* evidence *toward the affirmative.* "Does not apply" means that, in the case of individual patients, some items in function VI, application and execution of nursing procedures and techniques, and function VII, promotion of physical and emotional health by direction and teaching, may not be germane. "Evidence" means data on which a judgment or a conclusion can be based or on which proof or probability may be established.

Definitions of the subcomponents need to be studied, because they literally provide the base for examination of the chart in relation to the subcomponents and the functions to which they are attached. In the presentation of the definitions, scoring directions are omitted because scoring should be done by a trained clerk when the auditor has completed Part II by checking the box which indicates her judgment on each component.

# EXPLANATION OF AUDIT SCHEDULE COMPONENTS

## Function I. Application and Execution of Physician's Legal Orders

1. *Medical Diagnosis Complete.* The diagnosis is clear enough to permit intelligent execution of the nursing functions. A diagnosis

which conforms in terminology with that of the International Classification of Diseases, published by the U.S. Department of Health, Education, and Welfare, ordinarily suffices.[3]

At varying points in patient care, as when clinically unexplained changes occur, the maximum nursing base may be a tentative clinical diagnosis and other significant data that justify intervention.

Where patients have multiple diagnoses, the same rules apply. Here, one of the hazards in nursing and for the patient, however, is that the primary diagnosis in relation to which care is being given remains the sole focus of care, when the other diseases or disorders involved may be equally important in the nursing process. The patient who had cholecystitis with cholecystectomy, and also has longstanding diabetes mellitus, may receive much nursing attention for the surgical problem but only cursory attention to the problems he may have with regard to the diabetes.

2. *Orders Complete.* The physician's orders are clear, explicit, and conclusive *when looked at in regard to the patient, as well as to the diagnosis and other clinical data.* Orders for medications should include the dosage and frequency of administration and the route of administration (unless it is clear from the nature of the medication, as for aspirin or insulin). Orders should be specific not only when medications are administered by the nurse, but also when self-administered by the patient or given by family members or other responsible persons.

3. *Orders Current.* Orders are up to date according to pertinent institutional or agency policy *and* nursing judgment. For example, an order for Seconal may fall within the stop-order policy limit. But if there is evidence that Seconal is causing untoward effects in the patient, the nurse will withhold the medication and consult the physician about the situation rather than adhere to policy only.

4. *Orders Promptly Executed.* The chart shows reasonable and appropriate timing between the giving of the order and compliance with it. There should be adherence to institutional or agency policy in regard to the dating of the orders, the recording of the time at which the orders are written, and the recording of the date and time of execution of the orders.

5. *Evidence That the Nurse Understood Cause and Effect.* The chart shows that the nurse knew what she was doing and why she was doing it. A nurse performing any service ordered by the physician is legally obligated to understand the cause and effect of that service before performing it. The nurse is required to understand not only the basis for and anticipated therapeutic results of performance, but also the possible side effects or other complications. It cannot be too strongly emphasized that the nurse's right to perform any function is

absolutely contingent upon her ability to understand underlying cause and anticipated effect, as well as upon the ability to perform the function.

6. *Evidence That the Nurse Took the Health History into Account.* The chart reflects recognition that knowledge of pertinent points in the patient's past pattern of health and illness are vital to intelligent current nursing care.

The purpose of the history is to develop data from which to make nursing assessments of strengths, weaknesses, and life style which are taken into account when planning nursing intervention relative to health-illness problems.

## Function II. Observation of Symptoms and Reactions

7. *Related to the Course of the Above Disease in General.* There is evidence that the nurse understands the disease in the textbook or classic sense and is observing the patient with the classic picture as her clinical frame of reference.

By this is meant that the natural history of the disease from which the patient suffers should be known by the nurse and used as the clinical base for developing the nursing process. In this regard, the paradigm developed by Leavell and Clark is useful because it depicts the pattern of movement through prepathogenesis, early pathogenesis, discernible early disease, advanced disease, and convalescence, with possible outcome of recovery, a chronic state, disability, or death.[4]

8. *Related to the Course of the Above Disease in This Patient.* There is evidence that, in addition to the knowledge of the disease in item 7, there are observations of the patient's individual response to the disease and its treatment.

This simply means progression from consideration of the natural history of the disease in any man and the natural history of the disease in the particular man, which may be influenced by his heredity, his general health, and his life situation, as well as by his treatment and response to treatment.

9. *Related Complications Due to Therapy (Each Medication and Each Treatment).* Recorded observations relate to expected therapeutic and possible or unexpected untoward side effects.

The observations are one reflection of the nurse's ability to understand cause and effect relationships in nursing management.

10. *Vital Signs.* When indicated by the patient's situation, recording includes: temperature; quality of pulse, as well as rhythm and

rate; quality of respirations, as well as rate; blood pressure; tone, temperature, and color of the skin; and observations pertinent to feeling tone—that is, the patient's affective state.

Here the emphasis is on collection of data so that patterns and trends in the vital signs are clear. The recording of a single vital sign, such as one blood pressure determination, is meaningless because it is the trend in blood pressures that indicates need for, and response to, therapy.

11. *Patient to His Condition.* There is evidence that attention was given to the patient's attitude toward his clinical condition and life situation as it influences, and is influenced by, the clinical condition.

"Attention" means careful consideration of behaviors reflective of attitude. This includes use of direct, indirect, and reflective questions to the patient aimed at eliciting attitudinal responses, as well as observation of nonverbal behavior.

12. *Patient to His Course of Disease.* There is evidence that attention was given to the demonstrable degree of the patient's understanding and acceptance, rejection, or ambivalence toward his specific disease and illness.

Attention here is literally twofold: attention to the disease that is the pathologic process; and attention to the illness that is the acute or chronic manifestations of the pathologic process. For example, it is possible for a patient to reject his disease but to accept the illness it causes, or to accept the disease but reject his illness. Nursing intervention carried out without recognition of the patient's position will fall short of its mark.

## Function III. Supervision of the Patient

13. *Evidence That Initial Nursing Diagnosis Was Made.* The chart shows that nursing problems were determined and categorized as the basis for nursing care plans directed toward solution of the problems. This diagnosis should be made as soon as possible after the first nursing contact with the patient. In some charts, nursing care plans strongly suggest that a diagnosis was made. In this event, evidence of the implicit diagnosis should be taken into account.

Since "to determine" means to establish after consideration, investigation, or calculation, and "to categorize" means to classify into specified divisions, it is obvious that initial "nursing diagnosis" as here used encompasses the steps in the nursing process up to the point of formulation of the plan of care.

14. *Safety of the Patient.* There is recorded evidence of precautions taken to prevent physical injury.

These precautions include assistance in early ambulation and other activities involving neuromuscular functions which are difficult for the patient and encompass environmental safeguards as well.

15. *Security of the Patient.* There is evidence of work that helps in maintaining a therapeutic environment for the patient.

This work includes support of productive interpersonal relationships, as well as attention to the physical setting in which the human interactions occur.

16. *Adaptation (Support of Patient in Reactions to Condition and Care).* There is evidence of attempts to help the patient adjust to his changing condition, to the course of his illness, to his care, and to his anticipated future.

These attempts include helping the patient to accept attainable therapeutic goals; helping reduce the patient's anxiety, fear, and doubt; helping him toward self confidence and confidence in his care; and helping the patient to exert the physical and emotional efforts required in his situation, in accordance with his capacities.

17. *Continuing Assessment of Patient's Condition and Capacity.* The chart reflects ongoing evaluation of the current status and situation of the patient and the effects of care, with analysis of current nursing problems.

This continuing assessment involves both the collection of data with validation of them and interpretation of that data with validation of the interpretation as a base for modification or revision of the plan of care.

18. *Nursing Care Plans Changed in Accordance with Assessment.* There is evidence that the plan of care was adapted as nursing problems were altered by changes in the patient's condition and capacity.

In relation to assessment, the difference between this and item 17 is that item 17 emphasized continuity of assessment, as opposed to assessment of one or another single aspect of the patient's condition or capacity.

This subcomponent, however, is primarily addressed to the question of whether the nursing care plan was appropriately altered as the patient's condition and capacity changed.

19. *Interaction with the Family and with Other People Considered.* There is evidence of concern for the people in contact with the patient, with a view toward promoting interactions that are beneficial to all concerned.

This means that the patient's interactions with his family, his physician, and other people important to him are observed with respect to the interests and concerns reflected by them and use of those observations to advance mutually constructive relationships.

## Function IV. Supervision of Those Participating in Care (Except the Physician)

20. *Care Taught to Patient, Family, or Others Participating in His Care.* The chart reflects what care was taught, what guidance and support were given, to whom, and by whom accomplished.

The care taught includes all activities resumed or assumed by the patient and all the tasks performed by others involved in his care. It is assumed that care has not been taught until the behavior of those taught shows or suggests that learning has occurred.

21. *Physical, Mental, and Emotional Capacity to Learn Considered.* The evidence shows that the ability and readiness of those to be taught, guided, and supported were taken into account.

Consideration of the learners' capacity includes initial and continuing assessments of the need for and the appropriateness of that which is to be taught, in relation to the ability and the readiness of those being taught.

22. *Continuity of Supervision to Those Taught.* The evidence shows that the results of initial and additional teaching were assessed with appropriate follow-up.

This subcomponent is also based on the assumption of item 20 that teaching has not occurred until it is reflected in the behavior of the learners, and that activities and tasks in self-care or care given by others are not ordinarily learned through a single exposure to "teaching." The emphasis here is on the follow-up.

23. *Support of Those Giving Care.* The chart reflects the giving of emotional and physical help to those taught and supervised.

Here the emphasis is on continuing assessment of the ability and readiness of those taught, with appropriate action in accordance with the assessment.

## Function V. Reporting and Recording

24. *Facts on Which Further Care Depended Were Recorded.* The information recorded facilitated continuing physician and nurse management of clinical care.

Minimum information includes observations of symptoms and reactions; evidence of the execution of physician's orders; and data developed as part of the supervision of the patient.

25. *Essential Facts Reported to the Physician.* The chart shows that basic necessary information was conveyed to the physician either in writing or verbally. The facts may be major or minor; it is their importance to the physician and his management of the patient's care that makes them essential or nonessential.

Essential facts are those indispensible to patient-centered care, as well as those that are clinically significant as discrete facts.

26. *Reporting of Facts Included Evaluation Thereof.* There is evidence that, in reporting facts, nursing judgment concerning their significance or possible importance is included.

In other words, the emphasis here is on nursing expression of the reason why the facts were considered indispensible to the physician in the management of his patient.

27. *Patient and Family Alerted as to What to Report to the Physician.* There is evidence that patient or family members are directed to report to the physician those factors, signs, symptoms, or situations the direct reporting of which is conducive to patient and family rapport with the physician, or is otherwise mutually advantageous.

The intent here is to foster communications with the physician about questions which the nurse cannot properly answer, or questions the answering of which by the physician serves a special purpose in the management of medical or nursing care. One special purpose would be to have anxieties and fears allayed by the physician when he can best accomplish this.

Having the patient and family members report to the physician does not relieve the nurse of responsibility for direct reporting to the physician. In critical matters, the physician may be assisted by receiving separate communications from the patient or family and from the nurse.

28. *The Chart Permitted Continuity of Care.* The chart permits an uninterrupted sequence of care from nurse to nurse, from nurse to physician, and from nurse to other professionals. It is of major importance that the chart indicate succinctly that information vital to the patient's therapeutic regimen was reported to the physician.

The question to be answered in this subcomponent is not whether there actually was continuity in care, but whether continuity of care was possible with use of the information on the chart.

## Function VI. Application and Execution of Nursing Procedures and Techniques

29. *Administration of Medications/Supervision of Their Use.* Whether medications are given by the nurse, or whether the nurse is supervising the patient or the family in the taking or giving, the chart

reflects nurse or patient and family awareness of expected therapeutic results and possible untoward side effects.

For every medication, including those administered by the physician, there are anticipated therapeutic effects and possible untoward side effects, including reactions of intolerance and idiosyncrasy. Wherever more than one medication is used, the possibility of drug incompatability must also be considered.

30. *Personal Care (Bathing, Oral Hygiene, Skin, Nail, and Hair Care).* The chart indicates appropriate attention to personal care whether the care activities are performed by the patient, a family member, or another person.

Appropriate attention includes not only concern with cleanliness, but also with grooming conducive to feelings of well-being, personal worth, and dignity.

31. *Nutrition, Including Special Diets.* There is evidence of attention to adequate nutrition as appropriate to the patient's condition, course, and stage of growth and development. If a special diet is used, there is evidence as to whether or not, and to what extent, the diet and the main reasons for it appear to be understood and accepted by the patient and his family.

Appraisal of the patient's usual eating habits is a part of nursing assessment, whether the patient is on a regular or a special diet. Results are used in formulating and implementing nursing care plans.

32. *Fluid and Electrolyte Balance.* The chart reflects consideration of possible disturbances in body fluid and electrolyte balance, as indicated by the patient's age, condition, and course of illness.

Considerations of possible disturbances include attention to fluid intake and urinary output; changes in respiratory rate and depth; changes in skin turgor; dryness of skin and mucuous membranes; changes in behavior, such as increasing apathy or restlessness; thirst; ascites; and edema.

33. *Elimination.* Evidence that bowel function is considered, and that appropriate action is taken when the patient's bowels are not functioning normally for him.

The emphasis should be on what is normal for the patient in health and the derivations that occur because of his illness. Action should follow the patient's pattern as closely as permitted by his condition.

34. *Rest and Sleep.* Evidence that the patient's usual and unusual patterns of rest and sleep are taken into account in planning his regimen and supervising his care.

Appraisal of the patterns of rest and sleep is also a part of nursing assessment. It permits planning of the regimen with regard to rest and sleep, to follow as closely as possible the patient's natural rhythms. If the usual patterns obviously yield deficits in rest and sleep, the regimen should be planned with the aim of bringing about appropriate alterations of the pattern.

35. *Physical Activity.* The chart shows the relationship between the activity in which the patient engages and the activity which is clinically permissible. Where excess or deficit is found, efforts are made to reconcile actual physical activity with clinically estimated physical tolerance.

Development of a balance between too much and too little activity requires that the patient understand and accept the reasons that underlie restriction or increase in activity.

36. *Irrigations of Wounds, Canals, Cavities.* Evidence that irrigations are performed as ordered; the results; and, if dressings are used, what kind and whether sterile or clean.

This subcomponent refers to all types of irrigations and includes enemas. If problems in performance of the procedure arise either in relation to the irrigation or in relation to patient reaction to it, they should be recorded.

37. *Dressings and Bandages.* Evidence that these are applied as ordered or as indicated. Topical applications, if any, should be identified; the kind of dressing used and whether it was sterile or clean should be noted.

Observations of the wound site and adjacent tissues should be recorded in a manner that permits continuing appraisal of progress in healing and early detection of complications.

38. *Formal Exercise Program.* Indication that a treatment plan is carried out as ordered by the physician or as outlined by a physical therapist at the physician's request.

Here, the nurse is responsible for seeing that the program is carried on and also that supportive encouragement and assistance are given to the patient.

39. *Rehabilitation (Other than Formal Exercises).* Evidence of teaching or encouragement toward independent living—range of motion (ROM), active and passive exercises, activities of daily living (ADL), use of aids in ADL. If nursing rehabilitation is not required, there is evidence that the nursing care approach is restorative in nature.

Activities of daily living require motivation and participation in decision making which leads to the activities, as well as to the ability to perform them. Evaluation of the performance may increase or decrease motivation. At best, encouragement from the nurse reflects knowledge and understanding of this. The restorative approach has the same foundation. Activities of daily living include not only self-care but also other activities which give a positive meaning to the day for the patient.

40. *Prevention of Complications, Including Infections.* Evidence of work toward maintenance of hygiene, early detection of primary or secondary infections or other untoward symptoms; early detections of complications due to therapy; and prevention of avoidable disabilities, such as contractures.

Consideration of complications that might reasonably be expected, or prevented, is a part of initial and ongoing nursing assessment.

41. *Recreation and Diversion.* The chart indicates specific attention to the patient's need for activities which interest and amuse him and which divert his attention from disease and illness.

For counteracting disease- and illness-oriented tasks, activities, and limitations, the importance of recreation and diversion, however simple the related activities may be, cannot be overemphasized as part of orientation toward health.

42. *Clinical Procedures.* The chart shows results of urinalyses and other examinations done by nurses, if any; blood pressure determinations; and results of performance of other general nursing procedures.

43. *Special Treatments, Including Tracheostomy Management, Use of Oxygen, Colostomy Care, Gastric Feedings, Care of Decubiti, etc.* Evidence that the treatments were performed, indication of results, and evaluation thereof; observations pertinent to patient's physical and emotional reactions.

The preparation of the patient for the special treatment is a part of the performance of special treatments. Patient's preferences as to the way in which the procedure is to be performed should be recognized and adhered to, as well as possible. Where it is not safe to follow his preference, the record should indicate efforts to explain this and to enlist his cooperation.

44. *Procedures and Techniques Taught to Patient.* Evidence that any procedure or technique the patient can learn to carry out to his advantage is in fact taught.

This subcomponent is addressed to the development of increasing independence in self-care by the patient, within the limits of feasibility for him.

## Function VII. Promotion of Physical and Emotional Health by Direction and Teaching

45. *Plans for Medical Emergency.* Evidence that, by policy or by specific teaching, patient, family, and other personnel know what to

do in situations which are worrisome or dangerous for the patient and which arouse anxiety or fear in those responsible for his care.

Planning for medical emergencies is contingent on assessment of the emergencies that might reasonably be expected to arise, in terms of what the patient and his family perceive as constituting an emergency and what is clinically perceived as an emergent situation.

In accredited hospitals and nursing homes, there are specific policies for the management of major emergency situations. In auditing, it is necessary to note whether policies were carried out as necessary.

In public health nursing agencies, plans about what to do if medical emergencies arise are developed with patient and family and in conjunction with the physician, if the patient is under private medical care. If the patient is not under private care, the patient and his family should know precisely what clinical facility to use in an emergency, and how to use it.

46. *Emotional Support for the Patient.* Evidence of work toward helping the patient understand and accept his feelings about himself, his condition, and his care, and helping him develop his coping abilities and other potentials.

Provision of emotional support requires assessment of the special needs of the patient, his characteristic behaviors, and his psychosocial and cultural matrix. Without this data base, it is unlikely that the rapport and open communication necessary for providing emotional support will be achieved.

47. *Emotional Support for the Family.* The chart reflects impressions and facts about family reactions toward the patient and his condition, which can be used to help the family accept the patient's condition and their own feelings about it.

Providing emotional support for the family requires the same data base as that required in emotional support of the patient.

48. *Teaching Preventive Health Care.* Evidence of promoting and protecting the health of the patient and his family and of teaching about secondary prevention, that is, teaching the early detection of signs and symptoms which may indicate new disorders or complications due to established disease.

Assessment of the goals and motivation of the patient and family precedes discussion and use of selected educational tools with them. The teaching plan will be unique for the patient and his family, and its effectiveness dependent on the rapport already established. Minimally, patient and family need to understand the medical and nursing regimen and to understand, accept, and carry out the necessary procedures and activities.

49. *Evaluation of the Need for Additional Resources, Including Spiritual Guidance, Social Services, Occupational Therapy, or Continuity of Nursing Care Under Another Aegis; Homemaker Service.* Evidence that, when indicated, possible needs for consultation or direct service were assessed.

Evaluation of the need for use of additional resources should occur periodically throughout the time the patient is under care. Continuation care planning should be done well in advance of the patient's discharge.

50. *Action Taken in Regard to Needs Identified.* Evidence that nursing action was taken, with the knowledge of the patient's attending physician, for needs identified as relating to the promotion, by direction and teaching, of the patient's physical and emotional health.

It is of course useless to identify and categorize needs and problems unless action is taken directly or indirectly to help meet the needs and to solve or alleviate the problems.

# TRIAL RUNS

Discussion of the seven nursing functions, the 50 subcomponents, and the definitions should be followed by group examination of a single chart which reflects a total period of care not exceeding two weeks in length. Shorter charts are initially more difficult to audit, because the nursing process is ordinarily adapted to this time span of service. Longer stays yield discussion that is overlong for the purpose of practice definitions to 50 items.

If possible, the chart should be reproduced so that there is a copy for use by pairs of committee members. Where it can be done, it is helpful to type all narrative in order to eliminate the distractions caused by handwriting; graphic and other items can be in photocopy. This is the only time charts need to be reproduced, and is recommended here only to expedite this step in committee work.

If it is not feasible to reproduce the chart, then one member of the committe serves as the reader for the group after each member has scanned the chart.

The purpose of this exercise is to reach majority agreement on each of the 50 items. After discussion of evidence on some items, there is likely to be consensus; on others, there will be marked differences in judgment. Movement toward agreement is indicated when the differences in judgment lie between Yes and Uncertain, or No and Uncertain, on any given item. Where the difference is between Yes and No answers, there is need for special analysis of the evidence and the reasoning on which each of the responses is based. The group then weighs the evidence, evaluates the reasoning—and makes the decision.

It is unlikely and undesirable that there be unanimity in judgment on each of 50 items. Application of the criterion measures requires individual judgment of evidence. There are choices to be made in responses to each subcomponent, and the final overall judgment is set within a numerical *range* in acknowledgment of the impossibility of greater precision in appraisal.

If there is unanimity in judgment on every item, it is likely that one or two members of the committee are exerting undue influence on the group. The composition of a committee whose members are chosen on the basis of the recommended qualifications ordinarily precludes continuing domination by one or another member, although the group needs always to remain aware of the possibility.

During this exercise, individual philosophies about auditing and about patient care emerge and should be dealt with openly and constructively. Application of the definitions to the subcomponents in relation to the chart yields the first practical appraisal of and reactions to the audit instrument. General discussion of auditing is necessary, and it is useful as a preface to application.

Practice sessions in auditing continue after the first group exposure to the auditing. These sessions will vary in nature. For example, pairs of committee members can examine charts together; 10 or more charts can be examined, each committee member privately reviewing each chart; or charts can be examined in a variety of other ways. The practice sessions are then followed by critical group examination of the evaluations to establish interrater reliability, that is, whether judgments of the same charts by various examiners fall within the same numerical range on final scoring. This critical examination includes group analyses of all cases whose final scores reflect either excellent or unsafe care. This expedites the evaluation process.

Analysis of interrater reliability in scoring functional subcomponents is the next step. It begins with examination of the highest and lowest scores of each group of subcomponents and coninues until judgments for each subcomponent have been compared and rationalized, that is, made conformable within reason.

Interrater reliability has been established when any given patient care record privately reviewed by each committee member yields a common *overall* judgment of quality. That is, each member has come to the documented conclusion that quality in the particular case was Excellent, Good, Incomplete (good as far as it went, but it did not go far enough), Poor, or Unsafe. Agreement in judgment of each of the 50 components is not expected, nor is it necessary. There should, however, be agreement as to the quality of the execution of each function. Monitoring with regard to interrater reliability that begins in the orientation process should be carried on every three months as an on-going part of audit committee work, and is so presented in the orientation period.

The process of individual auditing and group discussion continues until the committee members are satisfied that they can rely on audit findings, and that the findings justify their satisfaction.

Experience in the orientation of audit committees suggests that the orientation can ordinarily be completed in 35 hours; more than 40 hours should not be needed.

There are many ways of expediting the process. One is to invest two or three days in a workshop. The workshop includes laboratory sessions in auditing and simulated committee work, with leadership which is knowledgeable about the method. Such a workshop can include representatives from several institutions and agencies. Workshops may be regional or statewide.

Workshops within an institution or an agency are frequently used as an introduction to the audit method. In this case, nurses who will not immediately serve on the audit committee could participate and obtain a view of auditing which they could then share with other staff members. But the workshops should be planned primarily as training sessions for committee members.

As usual, effective workshops require preplanning, with programming for success. Prospective audit committee members might be asked to take responsibility for planning and preparation. Particular attention should be given to the feasibility and desirability of circulating key materials for study by participants prior to the workshop. Charts should be prepared for use in the laboratory sessions. Facilities should comfortably accommodate the general workshop sessions and small group audit sessions. Resource people may or may not be used.

Another way is to have the committee enter immediately into orientation for their task. In this event, it is suggested that at least one, and preferably two, consecutive days be used for intensive work, with regularly scheduled three- or four-hour meetings thereafter.

Final decision as to the way in which audit committee orientation should be conducted in an institution or agency rests with the director of nursing service. Or, if several institutions and agencies are involved, decision rests with the directors as a group.

The role of the director of nursing service in relation to institutionalization of the audit is obviously a very important one. Auditing cannot be undertaken properly without her approval and support. It cannot be successfully developed as a standard procedure without her continued approval and support. Nor can action on the findings of the audit committee be implemented without her cooperation.

As has been said, the director should not be a regular member of the audit committee, but her participation in at least a part of the orientation process is essential.

By and large, the philosophy of patient care in the institution or agency tends to be a reflection of the director's philosophy. During orientation, the director has an unusual opportunity to consider her impact as reflected in audit committee discussions. Most directors wish to have, and should have, a working knowledge of the method to be used in quality assessment. Most directors welcome the opportunity to work with a task-oriented group of nurses who are not primarily concerned, at the moment, with questions of responsibility and privilege as ordinarily reflected by rank.

Experience with audit committees also suggests that the members value opportunities for an exposure to the director as a colleague concerned with the quality of care, rather than as "the director."

Plans for committee orientation, with or without a workshop involving other nurses, will depend on the climate of the institution and on the decision of how the process of change which the audit involves can be accomplished. It is not a waste of time to develop two sets of plans, to weight their respective merits, disadvantages, feasibility, and possibilities for success, and then to decide how the enterprise should be undertaken.

## Issues Emerge

To help in the all-important preplanning, it seems sensible here to mention some of the issues raised in all audit committee experience since 1952. Resolution of the issues should begin to occur early in the orientation phase of auditing; the need for this movement influences preplanning.

The first issue is that of the seven functions of nursing—one of which is "dependent" and six of which are "independent." As Lesnik and Anderson point out, the difficulty here lies in openly ascribing to professional nursing the authority for the independent performance of any act.[5]

In the performance of the dependent function, it is required that the nurse act under the order and the direction and/or supervision of a daily licensed physician, that she comprehend the cause and effect of the order, and that the order be legal.[5] She must also be able to carry out the order. The "direction and/or supervision" of the physician *relates to the order.* The execution of the dependent function obviously involves the exercise of nursing judgment. Further, unless the nurse is directly employed by the physician, the physician is ordinarily not liable for negligent performance by the nurse unless he had the opportunity directly to observe, or should have observed, the negligent act and refrained from taking action to avoid it.[5]

In other words, the dependence implicit in nursing's dependent function is considerably less than total. In addition, *the dependence is upon the order;* the dependent dimensions refer to orders. The direction and/or supervision of the physician relate to the order.

In the execution of nursing's independent functions, physicians' orders are not required. Physicians do not need to write orders for observation of symptoms and reactions, this being a function for which the nurse is in any event responsible. Physicians do write orders for selected observations to be made by the nurse, either because of special concern about selected critical aspects of care or, perhaps, lack of reliance on the clinical acumen of the nurse.

Application and execution of nursing procedures and techniques is an area in which the physician may order some of the procedures, such as the administration of medications, irrigations, and other special treatments. Here the nurse simultaneously carries dependent and independent functions. In view of the extent to which use of nursing judgment is necessary even to performance of the dependent function, the weight of responsibility for applying and executing nursing procedures rests with the nurse and on her judgment.

The issue of dependence and independence needs to be examined in relation to patients. In the first place, unless the nurse is directly employed by the physician, it is the patient, and not the nurse, who is under medical supervision. If nurses do not realize this and act accordingly in carrying out their functions, they are providing less than professional care for patients and are depriving physicians of a quality of collaboration in the care of the patients which they have every right to expect.

Secondly, delineation of certain nursing functions as dependent makes explicit the *responsibilities* of the nurse to the patient and to the physician. The *authority* of the nurse is and should be directly proportional to her responsibilities. Work toward resolution of the functions issue helps in dealing with another issue. This issue is whether nursing care should be patient-centered. Conceptually, this issue is not debatable; most nurses would agree in principle that care should be individualized. Discussions of the subcomponent definitions, however, reflect a range of differing opinions about both the desirability and the feasibility of care so oriented.

Among questions related to desirability are the following:

Should the nurse really talk with patients about their feelings about their disease and illness? Their care? Their hopes? Their fears? Their resources? What they see as their needs? Should the nurse make and record observations of patient behavior beyond those pertinent to the disease which led the patient to seek care? Family relationships as these affect the patient and his care, and vice versa? Should the nurse assess patient and family knowledge about disease, illness, and health promotion in relation to the present and possible future of the patient? Should the patient really be a partner in his care?

Questions related to feasibility include such points as the following:

We're so busy, how can we take the time to interact with the patient? How can we get to know patients during short periods of care? Won't physicians object if nurses talk with patients about themselves, their diseases, and their care? Will undue friendliness or familiarity develop? Shouldn't the atmosphere (in the hospital) remain impersonal? Won't physicians resent nursing assessment? Won't patients get out of control if we consult them about their preferences? Wouldn't we need more nursing staff if we individualized care?

Questions that deal with the desirability of patient-centered care can be discussed most productively during the performance of audits, in relation to the specific patients whose care is under appraisal. Some of the charts will clearly reflect deficits to which the audit committee, operating as the professional conscience of the agency, cannot subscribe.

Questions of feasibility center primarily on the organization of nursing service for delivery of care and on physician-nurse relationships.

In the organization of service, it is recognized that it is logistically easier to plan for tasks-and-activities nursing than to gear up a fuller nursing process within which tasks and activities then have their considered place. Mounting demands for care, rising costs of care, imputed shortage of nursing personnel, and increasing use of computer programming for efficiency result in strong pressures for care that is organized on the task and activity basis. If these pressures are permitted by nurses to prevail, then patient-centered care becomes an idle phrase and not a philosophy which controls nursing practice. Had there been evaluations, by whatever method, of the quality of the process of care, evaluations that yielded hard data for use in planning and developing better patterns of nursing care, the problems of providing patient-centered care would not be as grave as they now are.

The problem of physician-nurse relationships appears to be due to a combination of factors. One is the lack of clear and common definitions of nursing functions. Another relates to nursing's apprenticeship origin and to its relatively recent emergence as a profession that is both somewhat aggressive and somewhat defensive in its relations with physicians. Yet another factor for some physicians and some nurses is adherence to tradition and custom, simply because it is comfortable to walk well-trodden paths. Use of the nursing audit may be one small step on a new road.

Systematic efforts to measure and improve the quality of nursing care through auditing contributes to the overall improvement of care by focusing care on the patient and his needs and by clarifying the functions of nursing in relation *to the patient.* High on the list of the patient's needs is his need for collaboration between physician and nurse. If the physician-nurse collaboration is lacking, the patient's care is compromised.

A number of issues which arise center on institutional or agency policies which, in turn, are reflections of philosophy. In hospitals, one policy issue is use of the Kardex. The common practice is to set up the nursing assessment and care plan on the Kardex and to update the plan daily, with erasure of previous care items on the card. Upon discharge of the patient, the Kardex is destroyed, although some head nurses retain the Kardex when rehospitalization of the patient is anticipated. Entries on patients' charts are limited to the minimum amount of recording that is judged essential.

Use of the Kardex is evidence of concern for patient-centered nursing care, somewhat offset by concern for efficiency. For example, the Kardex is readily available, whereas the chart, which is used by physicians and others, often is not. Erasing the previous day's entries does, it is true, limit accumulation of recordings; but a patient's Kardex is not customarily reviewed by his physician.

The chart remains as the permanent legal record of care, and it is audited as such. The Kardex, however, reflects the process of care, at least on a one-day basis. It would be wise to retain the Kardex until auditing has been completed, for whatever help it might give the examiner.

The Kardex as ordinarily used, however, suggests some nursing inconsistencies. It is generally agreed that the patient's health history is germane to current care. Yet, the record of history being made during each hospital day by patient and nurse, as shown in the Kardex, is systematically destroyed, and continuity of care may thereby be impaired. If the physician does not regularly see the Kardex as well as the chart, he gets a limited view of the nursing care actually being given to his patient and of the rationale for the care. He may generalize from the limited view.

When the Kardex is talked about, it is justified on the grounds that nursing notes on the chart would be voluminous without it, and the bulk of the chart would be inconvenient both during the stay and later when the chart is filed with medical records after discharge. It should be noted, too, that in some hospitals nursing notes are not retained as part of the chart, but are destroyed. This then destroys the possibility of nursing care continuity for patients who are discharged with plans for nursing care to be provided by a public health nursing agency or by a nursing home. In this event, need for communication between the hospital nurse and a nurse in another facility may arise and may be critical for the patient. Continuity in nursing care for patients readmitted to the hospital at a later time is of course impossible if the nursing notes for the previous stay have been destroyed.

In public health agencies, the policy of writing nursing care plans is in general effect. This is so because of pressures from payment agencies and because of the agencies' belief in planning care around the needs of patients. Many of these plans, however, are primarily a listing of nursing tasks and activities, and are not planning of the nature inherent in proper use of the nursing process. In these agencies, too, efficiency in recording, with emphasis on control of volume, is an important objective.

In some institutional and agency settings, problem-oriented recording has been introduced;[6] a focus on problem-oriented nursing may ensue.[7] These approaches do not materially affect auditing and certainly do not alter the need for it. No evidence has been found to suggest that problem-oriented recording expedites auditing. This is not surprising because auditing requires clinical judgment of evidence, no matter in what form that evidence is arranged. Indeed, it is interesting to speculate as to whether problem-oriented recording reflects improvement in quality of care. Comparative audits using problem-oriented and traditional records might assist in considering the matter.

Overall attitudes toward evaluation in our society and in nursing need to be examined. Current use of evaluation tends to result in:

Anxiety instead of anticipation
Resentment instead of reward
Defeatism instead of encouragement
Compliance instead of self-determination
Safety instead of risk-taking[8]

Use of formative evaluation leads to positive attitudes and behaviors. Formative evaluation is that which refers to progress toward achievement of significant goals and objectives, and it occurs over time.[8] The nursing audit is designed as formative evaluation, and when properly used, yields positive attitudes accompanied by professional excitement and stimulation toward attainment of higher goals in nursing service by revealing ways in which the goals may be reached. Recognition of the basic formative nature of the audit as an evaluation mechanism usually occurs about midway in the orientation process.

During the orientation period, many other issues arise. The ones which have been mentioned here are basic and recurrent. By the end of the orientation period, the audit committee should have begun to deal with issues on the basis of priority. By that time, the audit committee members should have developed an understanding of the responsibilities inherent in their service as the professional conscience of the institution or agency in which they function.

The responsibilities of the committee, carried over time, center on measurement of the quality of care provided for patients, with resultant commendations for high quality care and recommendations for improvement in policy and practice, when necessary. The audit committee can be a major nursing influence leading toward provision of patient-centered care because it produces quantified data about quality that can be displayed and analyzed.

## References

1. Bloom BS (ed): Taxonomy of Educational Objectives, Handbook I: Cognitive Domain. New York, Longman, Green, 1956, pp 201–07
2. Krathwohl DR, Bloom BS, Masia BB: Taxonomy of Educational Objectives, Handbook II: Affective Domain. New York, David McKay, 1964, pp 176–85
3. International Classification of Diseases Adapted, 8th rev. U.S. Public Health Service Publication No. 1693, Washington, D.C., Government Printing Office, 1967
4. Leavell HR, Clark EG: Preventive Medicine for the Doctor in His Community. New York, McGraw-Hall, Blakiston Division, 1965, pp 15–19
5. Lesnik MJ, Anderson BE: Nursing Practice and the Law, 2nd ed. Philadelphia, Lippincott, 1955, pp 260, 277, 282

6.  Weed LL: Medical Records, Medical Education, and Patient Care. Cleveland, The Press of Case Western Reserve University, 1970, pp 13–14
7.  Woolley FR, Warnick MW, Kane RL, Dyer ED: Problem-oriented Nursing. New York, Springer, 1974, pp 1–6
8.  Reilly DE: Behavioral Objectives in Nursing Education: Evaluation of Learning Attainment. New York, Appleton, 1975, pp 90–91

# Chapter 8
# THE AUDIT COMMITTEE IN ACTION

The audit committee goes into action as soon as its members demonstrate, to their own satisfaction and the satisfaction of the director of nursing service, their readiness to assume committee responsibilities. Auditing is a committee responsibility; members are accountable to the committee as a whole. This fact helps the members who have developed beginning skills in the use of the audit instrument to assume their responsibilities as individuals, secure in the knowledge that the auditing they do will be judged by their peers. The committee maintains records of its proceedings.

The chairman of the committee will have been appointed after being selected in whatever fashion leadership appointments are made in the institution or agency. The appointment of the chairman and of the members should be confirmed in writing by the director of nursing service and acknowledged by the recipients. It might be well to consider appointment of an assistant chairman to assure continuity in leadership service throughout the year should the chairman be unable to carry out her functions at one time or another.

One of the first tasks of the committee is to estimate and plan for the volume of work to be done. The size of the committee will have been determined and, if necessary, modified on the basis of the number of cases to be audited each month. As has been said, no more than 10 cases per month should be assigned to each member.

If no more than 50 patients are discharged per month, all cases should be audited. If more than 50 cases are discharged, a 10 percent randomized sample of all cases discharged will suffice. A table of random numbers and directions for its use in case selection will be found on page 188.

It is of major importance that the cases to be audited be drawn, as a randomized sample, from *all* discharges, and not discharges from a given unit in the institution. The committee is charged with assessing the quality of care provided by the institution as a whole. Therefore, until auditing is firmly established as a productive standard procedure, and is so accepted by the majority of the nurses, auditing of cases from specific units within an institution or agency should not be undertaken.

The volume of work to be done is then related to the time required to do it in. The following example of time required for the auditing of 50 cases per month by a five-nurse audit committee may serve as a guide for committee planning.

The chairman assigns 10 cases to each member, including herself. The listing of the cases, with the name of the nurse to whom each case is assigned and date of assignment, is prepared by a clerk working under instructions of the chairman. The clerk also completes Part I, Hospital and Nursing Home Audit, or Part I, Public Health Nursing Audit. This should be accomplished in one-half day of clerical time.

The audit committee members are advised by the clerk that the charts are available. Each member then reviews the charts during working hours, at her convenience. It is well to restrict auditing to one area of the institution to prevent dispersion and possible loss of charts, and kibitzing by nonauditors.

When auditing skills are well developed, the time required for auditing averages 15 minutes per case for cases in which length of stay was three months or less.

Each member therefore invests two and a half hours each month in auditing the 10 cases—completing Part II, Nursing Audit Chart Review Schedule, and Part III, Audit Results, in each instance.

Cases that present problems to the auditor or that demonstrate exceptional (good or bad) quality dimensions are listed. These cases are presented to the committee for reexamination.

Each auditor is responsible for charts assigned to her until they are returned to appropriate custody.

The clerk does the scoring on the cases and enters the scores on Part III of the schedule. This requires approximately three hours of clerical time. The auditor reviews the scoring and signs Part III of the audit, at some time prior to the committee meeting.

When all cases have been audited, the chairman convenes the committee. During this meeting, cases presented by members are reviewed; moot cases are decided by congruence with theory *and* consensus: findings on all cases are reviewed; and the report and recommendations for the director of nursing are prepared and submitted, over the signature of the chairman. This work can ordinarily be accomplished in two or two and a half hours.

The clerk then types the report and a summary of basic identifying data from Part I of the audit schedules. A half-day of clerical time should suffice for the typing of the report and summary of basic data.

It should be noted that, if audit data are to be processed by computer, the clerk should be trained to prepare the data for the computer and then to prepare the statistical summary from the processed data.

Approximately 20 hours of nursing time and 10 hours of clerical time would, therefore, be required for monthly auditing of 50 charts.

Consideration of the nature of the report to the director of nursing, which includes a summary of audit findings, a summary of related basic data, and recommendations for the director of nursing service, is an early committee task even though reporting was discussed, at least in principle, during orientation.

The report includes the number of cases received and the number that were judged, overall, to reflect excellent, good, incomplete, poor, or unsafe care. It also presents an analysis of quality judgments with reference to the execution of each nursing function—that is, the number of cases in which quality in relation to each function is characterized as excellent, good, incomplete, poor, or unsafe.

In other words, the overall judgment is the generalization as to quality of the care given to patients. The particular judgments of each function show how the overall judgment was developed, and they specifically direct attention to areas of excellence which should be commended and those in which improvement should be made. That is, the particular judgments provide the base for action on results.

The nursing audit report form for the statistical summary which follows illustrates one way of organizing the summary data. *The directions for scoring each of the seven functions* apply, regardless of the format chosen by the committee for presentation of the summary.

A summary of basic data describing the audited cases should be attached to the statistical summary of the monthly audit. The data selected for the summary of Part I, Hospital or Nursing Home Audit, or Part I, Public Health Nursing Audit, should regularly include the following:

1. Distribution by age groupings. This permits consideration of growth and developmental needs of the patient population. The age groupings recommended are: under 1 year, 1 to 4, 5 to 14, 15 to 24, 25 to 34, 35 to 44, 45 to 54, 55 to 64, 65 to 74, and 75 or more years.
2. Grouping of cases by primary diagnostic category and the number of patients involved in each category. This gives some indication of the needs of the patients for care in relation to specific diseases and associated illness and disorders.

NURSING AUDIT REPORT _____  _____

               Month       Day           Year    /s/ Chairman, Nursing Audit
                                                                  Committee

_____

Name of Institution or Agency

NUMBER OF RECORDS REVIEWED [ ]

OVERALL EVALUATION BY      Excellent    Good   Incomplete  Poor  Unsafe
NUMBER OF CASES            [ ]       [ ]        [ ]     [ ]    [ ]

EVALUATION BY NURSING FUNCTION
AND NUMBER OF CASES

| | Excellent | Good | Incomplete | Poor | Unsafe | TOTAL |
|---|---|---|---|---|---|---|
| I. Application and execution of physician's legal orders | | | | | | |
| II. Observation of symptoms and reactions | | | | | | |
| III. Supervision of patient | | | | | | |
| IV. Supervision of those participation in care (except physician) | | | | | | |
| V. Reporting and recording | | | | | | |
| VI. Application and execution of nursing procedures and techniques | | | | | | |
| VII. Promotion of physical and emotional health by direction and teaching | | | | | | |

DIRECTIONS:

1. Overall results are summarized from Part III of completed audit schedules.

2. Results by function are summarized from Part II of completed audit schedules. For Functions I-V inclusive, use the final score attained; for Functions VI and VII, use the final score attained PLUS the respective "Does Not Apply" total. Relate the resulting to the judgment and
resulting scores to the judgment and the scoring range below.

| | | SCORING RANGE | | | |
|---|---|---|---|---|---|
| FUNCTION | Excellent | Good | Incomplete | Poor | Unsafe |
| I | (36-42) | (27-35) | (18-26) | (9-17) | (0-8) |
| II | (32-40) | (24-31) | (16-23) | (8-15) | (0-7) |
| III | (23-28) | (16-22) | (10-15) | (5- 9) | (0-4) |
| IV | (17-20) | (12-16) | ( 8-11) | (4- 7) | (0-3) |
| V | (17-20) | (12-16) | ( 8-11) | (4- 7) | (0-3) |
| VI | (27-32) | (21-26) | (14-20) | (7-13) | (0-6) |
| VII | (16-18) | (12-15) | ( 8-11) | (4- 7) | (0-3) |

3. Grouping of cases indicating the number of patients with more than one disease. That is to say, grouping by primary diagnosis and secondary diagnosis gives some indication of the complexity of the clinically required care.
4. Categorization of patients in accordance with the source of referral to the institution or agency. This focuses attention on the way patients entered the system and on admission policies, procedures, and practices. This categorization also, to some degree, shows how the community is using the facilities of the institution or agency. Sources of referral include:

Patient, family, friend                Hospital nursing department
Private physician                      Coordinated Home Care Program
Hospital clinic                        Neighborhood health clinic
Emergency room                         Other source (specify)
Hospital social service

5. Grouping of numbers of patients by discharge status. This provides an indication of some intermediate or final outcomes of care. These data are important for institutional or agency planning and evaluation of continuation care, and for analyses of the way institutional and agency facilities are utilized.
6. Discharge status. This includes discharges to self-care or family care; to public health agency care; to a nursing home: to other institutions (specify) or agencies (specify); discharges by death; and discharges to private physician care, with reference to self- or family-care.
7. Other categorizations which might yield information needed by the institution or agency for monitoring, planning, or evaluation purposes.

The last section of the report covers remarks and recommendations from the audit committee. The remarks include commendations for quality findings and other matters which warrant the attention of the director of nursing. The recommendations should be directed toward improvement of quality in clear, specific, constructive, and in brief terms. Rationales for the recommendations should be obvious or explained. In the judgment of the committee, action on the recommendations should be feasible.

If situations are found where there was danger to patients and a resultant need for corrective action or censure by the director, the situation should be summarized with identification of the persons involved. This is in no way a contradiction of the constructive nature of auditing. It is constructive to protect patients from harm; it is immoral to do less.

When the committee has planned accommodation to volume of work and is clear about the nature and purpose of the report to be submitted to the director of nursing at the end of each auditing period, the group then moves to establish institutional and agency nursing goals which are basic to the improved execution of the seven professional nursing functions in behalf of patients.

As has been said in a variety of ways, no institution or agency, or any part of either establishment, can properly set up its own basic standards for judging the quality of nursing care actually delivered to its patients, because the functions of the professional nurse are not altered by the setting in which care is given. Any lesser stance shows nursing not as a professionally effected process, but as a series of tasks and activities that may be defined by an institution or agency at its pleasure.

When auditing is undertaken, however, there is need to develop a statement of initial goals, then to revise the statement as those goals are reached and as experience reveals potentials translatable into new goals. Formulation of the initial and successive goals is a committee responsibility; the formulations become a part of the recommendations to the director of nursing service.

The goals will vary. They will depend on analyses of the answer to the question, "What is the quality of care provided?" This, of course, is the question the audit presumes to answer. The word "presume" here means assumed to be true in the absence of proof to the contrary. The goals will also vary according to the broader, ongoing institutional or agency efforts to improve quality of care. The audit should contribute to and strengthen the total efforts.

The goals should be expressed in terms of behaviors or actions proposed as desirable for nursing in the institution or agency, so that measurements can later be made of progress toward attainment of those goals. Five goals that illustrate this approach and, at the same time, reflect specific areas for needed improvement consistently found in all auditing experience to date, are suggested for consideration:

1. To extend the pathophysiologic basis for nursing care
2. To extend preventive nursing
3. To apply current knowledge of growth and development in the care of all people in all stages of health and illness
4. To apply current cause-effect knowledge to patients' medication regimens
5. To apply the concept of continuity in the nursing care of patients within the institution or agency (intramurally) and beyond institutional walls or agency boundaries (extramurally)

Extension of the pathophysiologic basis for nursing care includes assessment of the scientific foundation of the rationale for nursing care, acquisition of new knowledge, and application of the knowledge to the care of the patient.

One illustration of the application of a pathophysiologic basis for care begins with the question, "What are the physiologic hazards of bed rest to patients of any age?" Asher's answer is: "Rest in bed is anatomically, physically, and psychologically unsound. Look at the patient lying long in bed. What a pathetic picture he makes! The blood clotting in his veins, the lime draining from his bones, the seybala stacking up in his colon, the flesh rotting from his seat, the urine leaking from his distended bladder, and the spirit evaporating from his soul."[1]

This answer illustrates the breadth and depth of scientific knowledge required to plan and carry out the patient's care. This includes knowledge of anatomy, physiology, and human behavior. It includes knowledge of the pathologic processes that result in disorders, such as hypertension; phlebothrombosis, thrombophlebitis; atelectasis; pneumonia; nitrogen, calcium, and phosphorus imbalance; gastrointestinal tract dysfunctions; decubiti; and loss of self-image. This knowledge is essential to intelligent preventive, therapeutic, and supportive care, which require application of the concept of disuse phenomena and the related underlying concept of immobilization.

Carnevali and Brueckner have reassessed the concept of immobilization. They suggest that immobilization is "the prescribed or unavoidable restriction of movement in any area of the patient's life." They further suggest that immobilization be analyzed in terms of area (physical, emotional, intellectual, social); cause (disease, therapy, factors within the patient or his environment); direction (potential for change toward improvement or aggravation); sequelae (consequences, including side effects that may unnecessarily extend duration, or change direction of patient response); and volition (prescribed or unavoidable, desired or undesirable).[2]

In order to extend preventive nursing, it is necessary to understand the primary, secondary, and tertiary levels of prevention and their relevance to the nursing process.

According to Leavell and Clark, primary prevention includes disease prevention and health promotion—that is, prevention in the prepathogenesis period.[3]

Disease may be prevented by protection from exposure to harmful physical or chemical agents; protection from diseases due to nutritional deficiencies or excesses; protection from infectious diseases by immunizations; and protection from some noninfectious diseases through environmental controls.

Health promotion includes all efforts not directed at particular disease or trauma but, instead, toward the development and maintenance of a high level of wellness of individual, families, and other groups of people. It is therefore addressed to the healthy aspects the patient and his personality and to his health potentials. It includes attention to nutrition and weight; rest; sleep; recreation; pleasurable physical exercise in accordance with capacity; purposeful living in which there is commitment to values that give people feelings of worth, dignity, usefulness, and sense of belonging, and ability to cope with their situations. Much of health promotion is based on reasonableness, rather than on scientific knowledge that specific actions will individually or collectively enhance health.

All areas of concern in health promotion are of concern in the nursing process, even for patients in biologic crises, because nursing intervention is directed to the patient's health potentials.

Secondary prevention means the securing of prompt medical diagnosis and treatment of disease as a result of appropriate observations of symptoms and reactions within context of the patient's health-illness history, including heredity, which suggest possible predisposition to a given disease. Secondary prevention also includes the early recognition and management of complications due to disease and the prevention of iatrogenic disease. Iatrogenic disorders are organic or functional disorders related to treatment of other disorders or diseases, such as decubiti due to immobilization, or invalidism in a patient with heart disease when there is no organic basis for the limitation.

Tertiary prevention is rehabilitation. Nursing in rehabilitation has received much attention, and it appears that this level is more clearly and commonly identified than the other two levels. What does not appear so clear is nursing recognition that, frequently, tertiary prevention is required because secondary prevention was neglected. When that happens, rehabilitation becomes a salvage operation when shipwreck should not have occurred.

In preventive nursing, as in other areas of nursing, collaborative efforts between the physician and the nurse are necessary for the attainment by patients of the objectives implicit in prevention. And use of other resources may also be entailed.

Application of current knowledge about growth and development to the care of people of all ages, in various phases of health and illness, is essential to individualized care. As Beland points out, knowledge of the laws of growth is necessary to an understanding of human development; both the knowledge and the understanding are essential to nursing practice. Growth is a life-long process, quantitative, qualitative, and uneven in tempo. Rate and pattern can be influenced both from within and from without the body. Different parts of the body develop at different rates. Growth is unique to the individual, and it is complex.[4]

Throughout the life span, development is contingent upon growth and upon life experiences which sustain, impede, or advance the individual in achieving life tasks characteristic of his particular stage of development, and in fulfilling his potentials.

In auditing, evidence of concern with growth and development is most often found in the charts of young patients; the evidence seems to decrease with the increasing age of patients. It appears difficult for nurses to accept in operational terms the fact that self-actualization is a basic human need, regardless of the patient's age. The process of growth through which individuals seek to develop their human potentials is not bounded by time, and perhaps their human potentials are only translated by death.

Another factor that militates against depth in growth-and-development approach to patient care is the stereotype associated with designation of patients as "chronically ill." This labeling of patients seems to yield care that is disease-oriented. Too often, the care is directed toward symptoms the patient presents instead of toward the patient in his totality. An exception to this may be found in formal rehabilitation regimens which, at best, are holistically oriented to the patient and to his care with emphasis on his potentials as a person and with attention to the healthy aspects of his body and his personality.

When the stereotypes of "chronically ill" and "terminally ill" are combined for a given patient, personalization of care is impossible. There is a lack of understanding and belief in the patient's need for movement, change, and activity related to his environment, and there is the lack of the idea of moving forward through time toward a future containing purposes and goals. To these findings is added the assumption, or knowledge, that life itself will end in the presumably foreseeable future.[5]

Audit committees will get the full impact of the depersonalization of care as they see repeated evidence of the stereotyping which tends to obscure the individuality of human beings who suffer from long term disease or who are fatally ill. They will find increasingly distasteful the use of identifications such as "chronically ill," "terminally ill," or even "acutely ill," because these designations may inhibit or prevent the provision of intelligent, compassionate, and humane care. They will receive the full impact of how essential knowledge about growth and development is to nursing's armamentarium.

The application of current cause-effect knowledge in relation to patients' medication regimens becomes progressively critical. Regimens tend to be increasingly complex and to include an incredible number of newly developed preparations. On the other hand, familiarity with commonly used medications may result in contempt for them; that is, since their effects are well known and since they are often used, observations pertinent to their use are made casually or may not be made at all until the patient is far advanced in adverse reactions.

For every medication, including aspirin, there are anticipated therapeutic effects, limitations in dosage, contraindications, precautions, possible side effects, such as allergic reactions, intolerance, and incompatibility between medications. To these problems is added the tendency of patients to use medications not prescribed by physicians or not prescribed for the current episode of illness.

While patients are under nursing supervision, the nurse is responsible for having and applying current cause-effect knowledge of all medications administered to the patient. This is so whether the medications are self-administered, administered by the physician, by the nurse, or by others under the direction of the nurse. The nurse is also responsible for observing the patient with respect to the medication's effects and possible hazards, with a view toward prompt preventive or corrective actions. Daily, the development of patient medication histories grows more important; a nurse' collaboration with the pharmacist in this regard is as important as collaboration with the physician.

Planning intramural and extramural continuity of nursing care for patients who require it has received considerable attention in recent years. This is due in part to the concern of health professionals with continuity with care as a dimension of quality. Partly, too, it is due to the efforts of voluntary and governmental payment agencies, and other people concerned with reducing the costs of care, to have selected patients move from high-cost facilities to less expensive ones, as warranted by the patient's condition and situation. This is seen in the transfer of patients from one section of a hospital to another, from the hospital to their own homes, and in the transfer of patients from general short-stay hospitals to institutions of long-term care.

Experience with auditing, however, suggests that, where there is planning for continuity of care, the planning tends to be categorical in origin. Aged patients, "chronically ill" patients, "terminal" patients, patients who need formal rehabilitation regimens, and patients with certain diseases or disorders under special study, or who present special clinical problems are likely to be the focus for continuation care planning and action. Planning may also be categorical in relation to availability of payment for care, as might be the case with Blue Cross, Medicare, or Medicaid patients. Availability of payment is not, of course, a clinical criterion.

Planning for continuity af care between one part of an institution or agency and another should be simple. A summary of care and recommendations can be made a part of the patient's chart, as a requirement of the transfer process. It is rare to find this done.

Planning for extramural continuity of care involves planning with the attending physician. The nurse must make clear to him the rationale that resulted in planning for continuity of nursing care. And she must, with nurses in the follow-up institution or agency, be responsible for carrying on the patient's nursing care. Her planning includes transmission of a summary similar to the one used for intramural transfer of nursing responsibility.

Proper planning for continuity of nursing care entails evaluation of all patients to determine whether they have nursing problems which warrant continuity of care. It also requires consideration of resources needed to provide the care. If care in each instance has been patient-centered, the evaluation of even large groups of patients can be quickly accomplished.

Categorical approaches, such as concentration on the chronically ill, may result in failure to assess the problems of patients who do not fall into this category, but who may have major needs for continuity in care. Similarly, approaches to patients by income level or by age group may cause the continuation care requirements of patients who do not fit into these proper classifications to be overlooked.

Incidentally, "continuation care planning" is a designation that seems preferable to "discharge" planning. "Discharge" planning can easily come to be associated with the disposition of patients or the utilization of facilities, the use and costs of the facilities being the paramount considerations. Both associations lead to the depersonalization and devaluation of the patients, their problems, and their care.

The audit committee with a sound orientation, that develops a plan of work, gains experience in auditing, and establishes agreed upon goals, will emerge as a group characterized by strong identification by its members with its goals. The members will be capable of dealing with relevant issues, and they will be increasingly capable of influencing their internal and external environment in desired and desirable ways. The group will be developed as initiator and reinforcer of decisions about change for the better in the quality of patient care.

## References

1. Asher RAJ: The dangers of going to bed. Br Med J, December 15, 1947, p 967
2. Carnevali D, Brueckner S: Immobilization: reassessment of the concept. Am J Nurs 70: 1502–07, 1970

3.  Leavell HR, Clark EG: Preventive Medicine for the Doctor in His Community. New York, McGraw-Hill, Blakiston Division, 1965, pp 19–37
4.  Beland I: Clinical Nursing, 2nd ed. New York, Macmillan, 1970, pp 736–46
5.  Voerwoerdt A: Communications with the Fatally Ill. Springfield, Ill., Charles C Thomas, 1966, pp 3–16

# Chapter 9
## THE AUDIT COMMITTEE AND THE DIRECTOR OF NURSING SERVICE

The quality of the working relationships between the audit committee and the director of nursing service will be a major factor in determining the effectiveness of auditing as a formative element in relation to the quality of nursing care provided to patients in the institution or agency.

The audit committee exists because of the director's final decision that auditing is to become a part of the quality controls for which she is accountable. The committee is a new resource for the director. In the positive sense, working relationships are symbiotic in nature.

The committee:

Collects data pertinent to the quality of care being provided
Validates and interprets the data
Identifies achievements and needs that represent perceived relationships between the real and the ideal in quality
Determines need priorities
Formulates hypotheses about the relationships among observed phenomena
Translates the hypotheses into goals and related objectives
Makes recommendations for attainment of selective objectives to the director

The director:

Validates the recommendations in relation to overall quality controls
Develops a plan for action
Implements the plan
With the audit committee, evaluates the results . . .

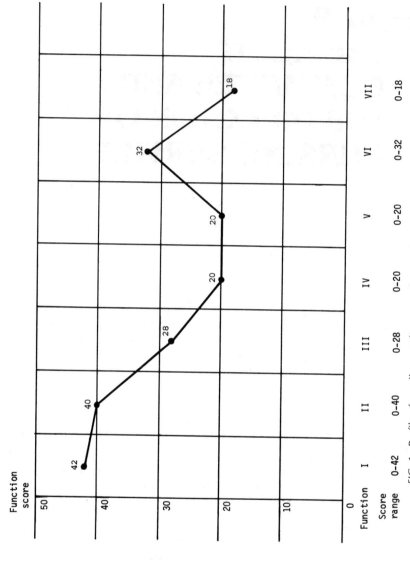

FIG. 1. Profile of excellence: Alignment of scores for seven nursing functions ideally executed; overall quality of care, score 200 (Excellent).

In these steps, the director follows through with the information and involvement of those persons and groups who were informed and involved prior to introduction of the audit as a standard procedure, and with others who have since become interested.

The audit committee should not be charged with responsibility for implementing the actions that it recommends. If that occurs, the committee as a whole, or some of its members, may lose their objectivity in auditing, and the objectivity of the committee may be challenged by others. It is obviously possible to be, or seem to be, unwittingly influenced by the desire to obtain favorable results from action that originated on one's own recommendations.

Because the committee is composed of nurses whose clinical competence is recognized, its members will necessarily be involved in changes that ensue from auditing. Their talents should be used, but they should not serve as the prime movers.

The committee and the director will find it useful to consider the profile of excellence that results from a graphic presentation of audit findings which reflect ideal overall quality of care and ideal execution of each of the seven nursing functions (Fig. 1). To have an explicit notion of the ideal helps in movement toward it. Systematic efforts to attain the ideal make it possible for today's ideal to become tomorrow's reality, leading in turn to more sophisticated ideals than those now projected.

The quality profile developed by the audit committee shows the committee and the director the answer to the question, "What was the quality of nursing care provided?"

Comparison of this profile with the profile of excellence helps the committee more quickly to formulate specific commendations and recommendations for improvement. It helps the director more quickly to analyze the committee formulations and to develop a plan for action upon them in the context of overall quality controls.

Figure 2 shows the profile developed after the first formal audit in the acute general hospital, in comparison to the profile of excellence. In the hospital audit, the overall score was 100; this score lies in the 81 to 120 range, which denotes quality as "incomplete." This means that the quality of care reflected in the charts was good up to a point, but that it had significant deficits either in scope or depth of execution of some or all of the nursing functions. In the comparison profile of excellence, the overall score was 200; this score lies at the top of the range for excellence, which is 161 to 200.

Quality profiles in institutions and agencies serve two purposes. First, they make clear the basis for *the generalization about the overall*

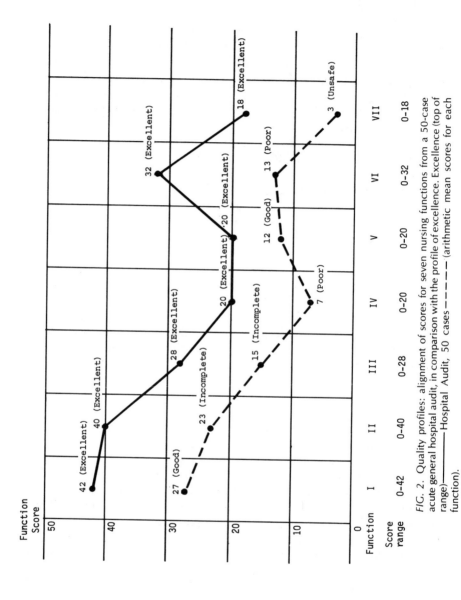

FIG. 2. Quality profiles: alignment of scores for seven nursing functions from a 50-case acute general hospital audit, in comparison with the profile of excellence. Excellence (top of range)———— Hospital Audit, 50 cases ———— (arithmetic mean scores for each function).

*quality of care* that was found on audit. The generalization usually tends to be encouraging, because in most accredited or certified institutions and agencies the overall quality will ordinarily be judged not lower than incomplete or poor. Unaccredited or uncertified facilities are not likely to use the audit method, unless they aspire to a higher level of community service than that which they currently provide.

Second, the profiles also make it clear that the cues and clues to strengths and weaknesses in quality are to be drawn from *the generalizations pertinent to each of the nursing functions.*

In the hospital example given earlier, the audit committee and the director breathed sighs of relief because of the generalization that the overall quality of care was "incomplete". They said, "That's not good enough, but we were afraid it would be worse." In other words, they were encouraged by the finding, though not made complacent.

These nurses then considered the generalizations about each nursing function and examined the subcomponents findings for each function to see where strengths and weaknesses lay. They decided that the strengths in execution of function I, application and execution of physician's legal orders, were availability of and access to medical diagnoses, completeness and currency of the orders, and promptness of execution. They found, though, that cause-and-effect knowledge was indifferently reflected, and that health histories were almost ignored, except for those pertinent to the present episode of illness. In function II, observation of symptoms and reactions, execution was seen as satisfactory, except for observations pertinent to the course of the diseases in particular patients and for data pertinent to patients' reactions to their conditions and the course of their disease.

The hospital credit committee further concluded that the execution of the other five nursing functions was seriously impaired by the weaknesses in the first two functional areas. The director's plan of action was geared toward phased improvement in the exercise of these functions, with involvement of head nurses and supervisors and, through them, involvement of staff. To all those participating in the nursing care of patients, the director conveyed her feelings of encouragement with the overall audit finding and her belief in the feasibility of improvement. It is equally important that she related the proposed changes to the goals of extending the pathophysiologic basis of nursing and of using knowledge about growth and development in the assessment of patients' nursing needs.

A major influence on the working relationship between the committee and the director are the feelings each has about audit findings, if feelings are shared. Experience with the audit in many set-tings suggests that nurses are perhaps so concerned with what they think is wrong that they take no pleasure from what is right. For this reason alone the sharing of feelings about the audit results is essen-tial.

Another necessary focus is on recognition of the qualitative im-provement of care that is brought about by use of the audit. Im-provement occurs over a span of time and should occur systematically in relation to audit goals. If this focus is agreed upon, then committee recommendations in each report will be relatively few, though well supported. And, because they are few, the director will be able to plan implementation. The recommendations should be cumulative in relation to audit goals so that, at the end of an audit year, movement toward attainment of audit goals is quite steadily reflected in succes-sive audit findings.

The audit committee and the director would be well advised to defer actions for improvement which entail participation of people not directly involved in nursing care until they have reasonable as-surance that actions are not being proposed to others until all possible nursing actions to correct a problem have been taken.

The wisdom of developing action with others is demonstrated in the following situation. On a first audit, the audit committee was in-clined to recommend putting pressure on physicians "to communi-cate better" with nurses about patients' medical regimens, including plans for discharge. The director was inclined to agree. It was de-cided, however, to defer the action until several audits had been per-formed. As it turned out, there was a prior problem about the ways nurses communicated with physicians. For instance, nurses did not discuss nursing assessments of patients with the physicians. Action then was first taken to encourage more open nurse communication with the physicians. Physicians responded well, and there was no need to put pressure on them. There did remain a need for some pro-cedural changes, which the nurses accomplished without exerting any power other than that of logic.

This illustrates one basic point. It is easier to address ourselves to the mote in our brother's eye than to the beam in our own. In audit-ing, it is particularly important to focus first on the nursing care and to see if nursing action upon nurses themselves will suffice. Only if it does not, should audit results be used to affect others who influence policy, procedures, and practice.

The audit committee and the director will be concerned about the attitudes of physicians to the nursing audit. This concern is entirely proper, even though the nursing authority to perform nursing audits cannot reasonably be open to question. The concern is a reflection of their realization that the patient depends on the physician and the nurse; that the physician and the nurse depend on each other; and that, when physician-nurse relationships are less than collaborative, the patient is the loser, while the professionals have a miserable time trying to work together. When there is poor collaboration, the environment becomes less than therapeutic for all concerned.

Physicians will be interested in nursing audits, because they have for approximately 20 years been familiar with the processes, outcomes, and problems of medical audits. It is interesting to note that some physicians who are developing new methods of conducting medical audits in service and educational settings are interested in the pathophysiologic and psychosocial components of nursing audits, as well as in the criterion measures used in them.

One constructive way for the audit committee and director to show concern with physician attitudes toward the nursing audit is to share the method and goals with interested physicians and to share findings, as appropriate, for the improvement of patient care and professional collaboration.

The administrators of hospitals, nursing homes, and public health agencies (other than the nursing director, if any) will be understandably interested in and supportive of nursing audits. The director of nursing service is responsible for interpreting the methods, goals, and findings to them. It is difficult to conceive of administrators who would be willing to say they are not interested in nursing measurements of the quality of nursing care, or who would obstruct the performance of audits. If this occurs, it is likely that the directors of nursing service are directors in name only.

There are four points on which the audit committee and the director must be in absolute agreement: (1) Completed audits *never* become a part of patients' charts. (2) There is *never* an indication on any chart that it has been audited. (3) Audit reports, together with the individual case audits on which the report is based, are filed with the director. (4) Minutes of all committee meetings are filed with the director.

The audit committee and the director should from time to time review the audit committee process to promote efficiency as well as effectiveness. The minutes and the audit reports provide the foundation for the review and for further planning and development pertinent to auditing as a part of quality control.

The time and effort required for auditing, and the resources needed for it, have already been indicated. One other resource is needed by the committee, the provision of which requires discussion with the director. That resource is the clinical and related references needed by the audit committee. The members of the committee will have at hand their own references of choice dealing with their clinical specialities or interests. They should also have access to current medical, as well as nursing and other professional, journals—and authoritative new books.

In addition, four basic references are suggested for use by the committee:

American Society of Hospital Pharmacists. American Hospital Formulary Service, Vols. I and II. Washington, D.C., American Society of Hospital Pharmacists, 1970

Beland IL: Clinical Nursing: Pathophysiological and Psychosocial Approaches, 3rd ed. New York, Macmillan, 1975

Benenson AS: Control of Communicable Diseases in Man. 12th ed. New York, American Public Health Association, 1975

Riehl JP, Roy C: Conceptual Models for Nursing Practice. New York, Appleton, 1974

The working relationship between the audit committee and the director requires a fine respect for their individual and joint responsibilities. The relationship is simplified and facilitated by the member of the audit committee who represents the director; this in no way lessens the need for optimum and direct working relationships between committee and the director herself.

All concerned must understand that, basically, no one likes standards except those of his own devising, and even these he wishes to waive on occasion, at his pleasure. Therefore nurses who are charged with responsibility for upholding standards of nursing care have particular need for good working relationships within which all major judgments of quality and their underlying rationales, together with resulting proposals for change, can be freely examined among the committee members and the director. It is especially important that a good relationship be established prior to action involving people who have not participated in the evaluation process, and who may not be as far along as the committee and the director in accepting the propriety of qualitative measurements of care through auditing.

# Chapter **10**
# THE INFLUENCE OF AUDITS

Audits accomplished by the method under discussion here do influence the concept, process, and content of nursing in institutions and agencies. They provide a basis for planning and developing nursing service with reference to quality of care provided to patients, and to quality control.

This is apparent in advanced workshops which are held some months after introductory workshops. In advanced workshops, participants acquire experience in auditing within their own institutions and agencies. The influence of auditing gradually becomes clear in the numerous, sequential sets of audit committee reports and minutes which are shared for the purpose of continuity in consultation and as a contribution to this book on the audit method. The following analysis of the influence of the audit has been developed primarily from these materials.

The fundamental conceptual change that occurs, upon which other changes depend, is a broadening of the concept of nursing. The seven functions of nursing come to be identified as seven ideas that, united, yield an enlarged general idea, or concept, which is identified as nursing. The broadened concept replaces a narrower concept of nursing based on the ideological union of three functions: that is, carrying out physicians' orders, observing acute symptoms and reactions, and performing nursing procedures.

To say that the broadened concept of nursing is born of auditing would be as presumptuous as it is untrue. Most nurses would, in principle, subscribe to the broadened concept without any familiarity with a nursing audit. The contribution of auditing lies in its crystallization of the subcomponents essential to the performance of each function and its emphasis on the fact that, in terms of each patient, the whole of nursing is greater than the sum of its separate functions.

Theoretical reexamination of the nursing process by the audit committee is a natural outgrowth of the broadened basic concept of nursing. All audits to date have shown that: (1) The best executed function of nursing is the carrying out of physicians' orders, (2) nursing care plans tend to be a listing of nursing actions to be taken; and (3) the actions tend to be task- and procedure-oriented rather than patient-oriented. Early in auditing experience, it is usually found that current chart formats are not conducive to goal-oriented nursing.

Audit committee recommendations usually lead to agreement about the nursing process model to be used under the leadership of head nurses and supervisors, in conjunction with staff nurses. Whatever model is chosen, there is emphasis in the recommendations on initial and continuing assessment of the needs of patients as perceived by *nurse and patient* with a *reconciliation of their perceptions;* on nursing action designed on a scientific basis to bring about desired changes in patient behavior, with his participation; and on validation of the nursing actions.

The development of an agreement about the nursing process model is achieved in various ways. One is the use of case conferences, another is the use of formal and informal group discussions with or without supervisory leadership. In-service education programs are yet another; these programs should involve part-time as well as full-time nurses. Agreement might also be reached through the trial use of various models in volunteer units within the institution or agency.

One useful means of efficiently focusing on the nursing process is to have staff nurses use Part II, Nursing Audit Chart Review Schedule, as a guide in the care of patients for whom they are responsible. If the schedule is used in this manner, scoring is of course omitted because it cannot properly be done until the patient has been discharged. This use of the schedule was initially proposed by staff nurses in hospitals, nursing homes, and public health agencies; it was not foreseen when the audit was developed.

A more recent development that seems promising is the development of nursing care plan guides on the basis of the seven functions of nursing and their subcomponents, with provision for continuing reassessment of problems and goals.

Audits also show that health histories are not ordinarily taken and used by nurses, even though an essential understanding of the patient's health and illness in relation to his human condition cannot be attained without an historical perspective. The purpose of the history is to collect data about physiologic, emotional, mental, and social aspects of a patient's life pertinent to his care. Without use of his health history, the care of the patient cannot in a real way be personalized. Knowledge of the health history is an integral part of nursing assessment.

A movement by nurses to initiate use of health histories occurs early after a first experience with auditing, precisely because health histories help personalize care. The depersonalization of care is so painfully apparent after the audit review of charts that audit committees invariably are moved to recommend changes. Advancing even limited use of health histories is an immediate action that can be taken without much difficulty.

Problems in the personalizing of care, however, have deeper roots than omission of histories. The apprenticeship origin of nursing is still reflected in nursing's focus on the physical care of the patient. Audits prove that physical care is often even further subdivided into care directed to various organs, or to body systems, or even to surgical wounds. It is not insignificant that patients may be referred to as "the cardiac," "the diabetic," "the appendectomy," or "the amputee."

The problem of depersonalization is further compounded by a number of factors. The provision of physical care is easier than the provision of holistic care. The word "holistic" means "whole" or "entire." Philosophically—and this is the definition of choice—the meaning is that whole entities, as fundamental components of reality, have an existence other than as a mere sum of their parts. Holistic care requires involvement and interaction with patients. It entails thought and feeling, with expressions of them, as well as a recognition of the responsibility inherent in nursing's entry into the life of the patient. It requires knowledge of human behavior applied to involvement and interaction. And it takes time. In contrast to these requirements, physical care can be accomplished quite simply and technically by carrying out action on one or another part of the patient's body, with minimal interaction between nurse and patient.

Another factor leading toward depersonalization is the prevailing pattern of organization for delivering services, so that various care tasks can be swiftly carried out for large numbers of patients. It may be that assembly line methods of service geared to efficiency in "production," with patients going through the line in rapid succession, will become the normative standard of service, unless concerted nursing efforts are directed to giving top priority to effectiveness of care, allocating efficiency to second place. This simply means that true efficiency lies in meeting the goal of effectiveness with the minimum expenditure of time, effort, and resources.

This problem is compounded by the availability of third-party payment for care services on a tasks and activities basis, and the nonavailability of payment for the process of care (which is greater than the sum of its parts).

Audit committee reports recently received from public health agencies and nursing homes include statements to the effect that audits show that care is not so much being given in accordance with the nursing standards of the institution or agency, but in accordance with third-party payment regulations. Hospital audit reports reflect concern with the negative impact of hospital utilization controls on the continuity of nursing care. Decisions to discharge patients may be made only in relation to the end of the patients' *medical* needs, which would mean the end of third-party payment for continued hospital care. Adequate attention is not given the *nursing care* needs of patients, that require continuity either within the hospital or outside of it.

Audit committee reports include recommendations for corrective, or at least remedial, action as judged appropriate for the institution or agency. Selected audit findings are used as a hard data base to support the recommendations.

In general, audit committee recommendations include actions directed to the improvement of the content of nursing, with special reference to its scientific basis. That basis encompasses knowledge derived from the biologic, physical, and behavioral sciences as they are unified and adapted for use through the nursing process.

More attention is paid in the clinical content to the conditions most frequently seen in patients, such as common heart diseases, diabetes mellitus, and malignancies of various types, than to conditions rarely seen. Attention, however, is also paid to the rationales of the new modalities coming into use in treatment of common diseases. This focus of attention is logical, because the care of patients who have common diseases and illnesses can easily become routinized and, in a sense, automatic, even though the situation is unique for each patient.

Approaches to the appraisal and updating of clinical content vary among institutions and agencies. Some may concentrate on the content needed in the care of patients who are in varying degrees of congestive heart failure, who have neuromuscular disorders or problems in fluid and electrolyte balance, or who have diabetes mellitus as a primary or secondary diagnosis. The psychosocial aspects of care for patients in various stages of growth and development may be the clinical focus, particularly where audits show that physical care is the center of concern.

In institutions whose primary concern is care of the sick, the clinical content needed for the care of patients whose death is imminent inevitably becomes an area of concentration, for the depersonalization of these patients is too often total.

Use of the audit in specialty settings, such as psychiatric facilities, institutions for the mentally retarded, maternal and child health services, ambulatory services, and public health agencies in which the care of the sick is not a major function, has followed a general pattern. The pattern is to try to change the audit subcomponents; to alter numerical weightings of the functions and the subcomponents; or to use only a part of the audit schedule, such as three or four of the functions, instead of using the seven functions. In these situations, at best, there has been ensuing recognition that the nursing process—the execution of the seven functions—is basic to professional care regardless of the particular clinical situation. Content and emphasis may vary, but execution of all seven functions is essential to holistic nursing. In any setting, literal use of the definitions of the subcomponents puts the functions in a patient-oriented perspective.

In long-stay institutions, it has sometimes been necessary to designate a simulated discharge date, a cut-off point for auditing purposes, or to use the dates of transfer of patients to an acute care facility for diagnosis and treatment as discharge dates. The number of instances in which institutional care has been going on month after month or year after year without periodic assessment of patient problems and potentials underscores the need for auditing. It has happened that reassessment of patients after auditing has led to substantial change for the better through fresh nursing interventions. The case of the nursing home patient who was able to return to independent living in the community after six years of dependence in the nursing home illustrates the point in a way that disturbs complacency in the care of presumably helpless—and hopeless—human beings in whom there may yet be untapped potentials for living.

In auditing records of long-stay care, as elsewhere, the audit schedule including the numerical values assigned to the components and subcomponents cannot be modified without destroying the validity of the instrument. This is not to say that the audit should not be used in any sensible way for improvement of care. It is simply to say that modifications invalidate the use of audit findings for generalizations about the quality as portrayed in quantitative measures.

The methods used to develop a common model for the nursing process that is to be used or refined within an institution or agency are also used to enlarge clinical content. The goal is self-development by the nurses who participate in conferences, work-shops, and in-service education programs. Results are judged over time, from audit findings. The fact that they are to be judged in this manner influences the kind of learning experiences provided formally and informally at staff, supervisory, administrative, and combined levels. The quality measurement inherent in auditing seems to lead to more specific efforts to evaluate the usefulness of activities directed toward the improvement of care.

At best, three main ideas seem to influence both the auditing and the actions taken as a result of auditing. The first idea is that it is the patient and not the nurse who is under medical supervision. The sec-ond is that the open making of nursing judgments is not only proper but is also a categorical imperative in professional nursing. The third idea is that judgments should be based on data and rationales which are documented, if they are not self evident, and that they be open to examination leading to validation—or, perhaps, invalidation—by peers.

When these ideas are built into the intellectual disciplines of nursing, and are used primarily for the advancement of patient care, there is little need for nurses to be defensive or devious in their work-ing relationships with physicians. As the audit was developed, it was correctly assumed that most physicians, like most nurses, care about the patients they take care of and that they respect efforts to measure quality and to improve it. Except for the patient, no one benefits more from quality in nursing care than his physician.

Charts are an important means of communication between nurses and physicians. The chart is one of the instruments through which the physician develops his perceptions of nursing. Audit committees are well aware of this, and their dissatisfaction with the format and use of charts, in service to patients, is intensified by this awareness.

Charts currently employed in institutions and agencies now using the audit—at least, those reported on to this writer—are illogi-cal in concept and inefficient in format; they create obstacles to the nursing process, sometimes hindering collaboration with physicians.

One problem with charts is the notion that chart recording is "paper work" and that it is an indirect nursing activity, when in fact continuity of care and the safety of the patient depend on a recording of that care. Recording is therefore an integral part of one of the seven functions of nursing. It is not an "indirect" activity.

Chart formats impede the nursing process because they do not encourage development of the data base necessary for care. They fail to facilitate identification of problems from the patient's health history or to pinpoint the problems to which nursing will be addressed. Nor do they provide space for the initial plan of action for the selected problems and for progress notes that follow through to new problems or changes in plans, or discharge summary.

Work with the nursing audit has made it abundantly clear that quality nursing care entails the use of problem-oriented charts/records. Weed has come to the same conclusion about medical care. To his conceptualization of the problem-oriented record, he adds a flow sheet which contains all the moving parameters on all problems that show complex data and time relationships.[1]

It might be well for physicians and nurses to move more quickly toward a problem-oriented *patient care* record, rather than to limit efforts to "medical" and "nursing" records development.

Weed adds a flow sheet which contains all the moving parameters on all problems that show complex data and time relationships.[1] It is interesting that Weed includes "notes by nurses and paramedical personnel" in the medical progress notes.

An objection raised by nurses to recording the nursing process used in patient-centered care is the time it takes; if recording takes too much time, there will not be time enough left to give care. Another objection is that proper recording would take up too much space on the charts. The objection seems based on two assumptions. One is that effective recording is voluminous. This is not necessarily true; analysis of the needs of the patient, if thoughtfully made, may be briefly recorded, with selection of essential data, only, for entry on the chart. The other assumption seems to be that human beings are complex, and that the patient-centered approach takes time. There is no quarrel with this assumption. There are no simple interactions between human beings when one of them is a professional nurse responsible for the care of the other.

The first objection is a disturbing one because it implies that staffing patterns are primarily determined by the tasks and activities to be performed instead of being oriented toward the assessed nursing needs of patients.

The second objection also reflects a devaluation of nursing and of recording. This devaluation is confirmed when nursing notes are stripped from hospital charts and destroyed when the patients are discharged. In some hospitals when audits were done, legal counsel was questioned about the policy of discarding nursing notes, and advised that the policy be changed to retention, because nursing notes are evidence, the absence of which might contribute to successful malpractice or negligence suits against the hospital.

Two broader influences of a different nature have been noted.

The nursing audit is frequently used in nursing education as an added way of teaching the nursing process; that is, to cast the process in terms of the nursing functions and their subcomponents and, also, to relate this view of the process to the previously mentioned American Nurses' Association's standards for generic and specialty nursing practice. In some instances, this use of the audit has included introduction of the method in institutional nursing services. It should be emphasized that when the audit is used by students, the scoring mechanism should not be used except on groups of cases that are appraised by a properly prepared audit committee. It is encouraging to note that some students have been later responsible for introducing the audit in institutions and agencies whose staffs they joined after graduation.

The second influence is a beginning identification of the ways in which the audit method and results may be used in interpreting nursing and its work toward quality assurance with laymen—including lay members of boards of directors and some board committees in institutions and agencies. Such use does seem to help clarify the perennial questions, "What is nursing?" or "What do nurses do?" and to help develop positive attitudes toward nursing.

The audit has been similarly used with consumer groups of varying educational levels. On a trial basis, some lay persons have been participant observers in simulated audit committee sessions. Here, particular sensitivity to the personalizing or lack of personalizing of care was apparent, as was the expressed recognition that the scientific and technical aspects of care required professional appraisal. These experiences support the idea that consumers are interested in knowing what is being done to control quality; how it is being done; and that they are concerned with the rights of patients as human beings. When these interests are satisfied, there seems to be no desire to participate directly in the actual quality appraisal process. In any event, there are two primary concepts in which it is hoped most people would agree—the consumer, however defined, has the right to quality care, and that he ought to have knowledge of and something to say about the planning and development of quality assurance systems. The opportunity to learn about and have some opportunity to respond to one method was valued by the consumers who were offered a focus on the audit as one part of the larger whole of quality assurance.

On the whole, the audit exerts considerable influence on an institution or agency. That is so partly because it brings nursing into focus as a major component in patient care; for nurses and other people, this forces a new look at nursing responsibilities. Measurements of quality reveal commendable strengths. They also show up weaknesses which are correctable if the broad concept of nursing earns common acceptance and is applied in common practice.

## References

1.  Weed LL: Medical Records, Medical Education, and Patient Care. Cleveland, Ohio, The Press of Case Western Reserve University, 1970, pp 13–14

# Chapter 11
# SOME IMPACTS OF AUDITING

Final appraisal of the impact of auditing on the quality of nursing care is the responsibility of the director of nursing. The director and the audit committee, however, will appraise each audit report in the light of all preceding audits, and they will evaluate the auditing process as reflected in committee minutes.

After a year of monthly auditing, progress in the pursuit of quality should be apparent when comparisons are made between the findings of earlier and more recent audits.

The following illustrations of forward thrusts toward quality are of interest because of the trends they portray. Audit findings and the actions taken on them will vary among institutions and agencies. These establishments vary in their climates, potentials, and problems. The illustrations given are, therefore, not necessarily useful as respective exemplars for hospitals, public health agencies, or nursing homes.

In the acute general accredited hospital, whose randomized-sample, 50-case audit was previously cited (p. 96), the audit committee recommended that improved observations of symptoms and reactions be given priority as an area for concentrated efforts. The committee reasoned that, if observations of symptoms and reactions were improved, then development of care plans would also improve because the data base on which they partly depend would be extended.

The committee suggested that audit findings, priorities, and the reasons for them be discussed with the nursing administrative and supervisory staff, and with head nurses, and then be presented for discussion in regularly scheduled staff meetings. Discussions were to include planning for follow-up on the hospital floors by head nurses and staff, with supervisory assistance.

The committee further recommended that policy regarding use of the Kardex be changed from that of day-to-day erasure to maintenance of a running record retained at least until after auditing.

The director of nursing supported the recommendations and added two actions. The first was to use the audit committee as a resource group in the general staff meeting. The other was to have the head nurse of the intensive care unit, who was a member of the audit committee, serve throughout the hospital as a resource person to oversee the observation of symptoms and reactions of patients recently transferred from her unit to general care units. This head nurse was relatively new to the hospital and well prepared for her responsibilities. She had previously had little opportunity for interaction with nurses outside of her unit.

The director had another reason for this action. In six cases out of the 50-case audit, the auditors had indicated that, while the overall quality of care was either good or incomplete in these instances, it was the quality of care in the intensive care unit that had raised the total level. In other words, there was a drop in the quality of care after the patients were transferred to general care. The director reasoned that true continuity of care among the units was essential, and that it might be promoted by the use of the intensive care unit head nurse as a resource. The arrangement was more than satisfactory to the head nurse because she had been concerned about continuity and had not yet devised a strategy for action.

The director advised the administrator of the hospital, the medical directors of the various clinical services, and the patient care committee about the nursing action being taken, and why. The plan of action was favorably received.

Six months later, audit findings showed an improvement of the overall quality of care (Fig. 1). Other changes had occurred in the institution during those six months, to be sure. But the audit committee and the director discounted them as having a significant impact on the quality of care. At the six-month stage, the overall quality was rated as good. The score was 130.5, which falls in the range between 121 and 160. This is in contrast to the first overall rating of incomplete, with a final score 100, which lies in 81 to 120 range. The quality of observation of symptoms and reactions had moved from incomplete (23; range 16 to 23) to good (31; range 24 to 31). There was some improvement in all of the other categories.

It is noteworthy that, in this hospital, the first change undertaken after auditing was a relatively simple one. It dealt with a familiar and commonly accepted nursing function, about which all participants in

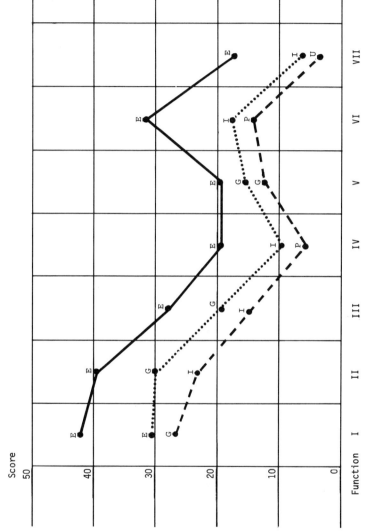

*FIG. 1.* Quality profiles: alignment of findings: acute general hospital. First audit, 50 cases; audit 6 months later, 50 cases; and comparison with profile of excellence. Excellence ————, First Audit — — — — —, Audit 6 months later . . . . . . , E Excellent, G Good, I Incomplete, P Poor, U Unsafe.

113

care have major concerns. It had a reasonable chance of success over time, but not instantly, and it was presented as advice to interested persons. (They, of course, were also pleased when the six-month graph was later presented to them.) In addition, the action taken by the director served administration purposes beyond an immediate quality purpose.

The statement that, during the six-month period, there occurred no other changes which were considered significant to the quality of nursing care warrants comment. The fact that the audit became a standard procedure does make explicit a new focus on quality and its appraisal, and this can affect the climate of nursing practice. In addition, other changes may have occurred in the hospital that did directly or indirectly contribute to improvement of quality. If auditing were carried on as a research operation, there would be a need to control, as much as feasible, the variables that could reasonably be expected to affect audit findings. However, auditing in institutions and agencies, conducted as a standard service operation, has as its goal the improvement of patient care. It is obviously not a research operation, but an attack on the problem of quality.

In an accredited public health agency, the first randomized sample audit of 32 cases indicated that the overall quality of care was incomplete, with a score of 95.5 (range 81 to 120). The two nursing functions where deficits were apparent were observations of symptoms and reactions (score, 15; range, 8 to 15) and execution of nursing procedures and techniques (score, 13; range, 7 to 13). In other words, there was poor quality of execution of both functions.

The audit committee recommended that the execution of nursing procedures and techniques be given attention by each supervisor, after local staff meetings in which the findings were discussed and the plan of action presented. The director agreed with this recommendation. She also suggested that attention be paid at the same time to observation of symptoms and reactions, because omissions in observation might be a contributing factor to the deficits in execution of all the nursing functions.

The majority of staff concurred with this view. They asked for copies of the chart review schedule to be used, without scoring, in analyzing their own case loads. They further asked that, when the analyses were completed, local in-service education conferences be held to consider results. In addition, at local centers where team nursing was practiced, team leaders used the analyses as part of their ongoing assessment of patient and family needs for nursing care and revision of care plans.

The audit committee members were asked to serve as discussion leaders in the various centers where they worked. After committee consideration of the request, it was declined, lest action by individual members, acting as leaders, be construed as the will of the committee. The supervisor member of the committee decided not to act as discussion leader in the conferences in her center, although she would ordinarily have taken this role. A senior staff member volunteered to carry the discussion leadership responsibilities; this proved satisfactory to all concerned. It is worth noting that the audit committee's reputation for objectivity was markedly enhanced by these decisions.

When the pooled problems relating to the execution of the two functions were examined, the following deficits appeared.

1. Nurses had not previously felt responsible for observation of expected therapeutic and possible untoward results of medications other than those they themselves administered. Medications self-administered by the patients were not labeled by name; and inquiry had not been routinely made of physicians with regard to medications they administered.

2. Several patients were taking medications not prescribed by the physician now responsible for their care. In one instance, a patient was taking tranquilizers previously ordered as well as those currently ordered. The patient was depressed and resisted the physician's recommendation for psychiatric appraisal. After the nurse discovered the duplication of medication and discussed it with the physician, the patient's total regimen was revised and tranquilizers were omitted altogether. The patient became more responsive in about two weeks and agreed to psychiatric care.

3. Nursing attention seemed to be focused more on various manifestations of disease than on the patients as individuals. In addition, patients' usual patterns of rest, sleep, and exercise were not taken into account in a meaningful way. One team concerned itself with assessing their patients' daily activities and found that the patients' daily lives revolved around their illnesses in a manner not warranted by the clinical conditions. It was the team's conclusion that nursing had contributed to this state of affairs; the team reoriented nursing care with results that were satisfying to themselves as nurses, as well as to the patients and families.

4. In this agency, blood pressure determinations were made only when ordered by the physician. Even though a number of patients were known to have hypertension, the taking of blood pressures by nurses was rarely ordered. The Medical Advisory Committee was consulted and after several sessions agreed that, since blood pres-

sures are vital signs, and the observation of vital signs is a part of nursing responsibility, the taking of blood pressures did not require physician order. The committee decision was a majority one and was made partly because one physician had a patient who was monitoring his own blood pressure. It was therefore considered particularly illogical to deny the right of a nurse to assess this vital sign.

5. Family members were being viewed primarily as resources in the care of the patient, with relatively little attention to their own health and well-being except as this might affect the care of the patient. To focus nursing attention on the health needs of each member of the family, use of individual record sheets was instituted as a part of the family record. The individual records are also essential in auditing. The in-service education program was planned to explain the concept of "the family as the unit of service" and its application in nursing practice.

As shown in Figure 2, the audit conducted six months later showed that the overall quality of care had risen to good, with a score of 124.8 (range, 120 to 160). Performance in the execution of nursing procedures and techniques had risen to incomplete, with a score of 17 (range, 14 to 20). Observation of symptoms and reactions had reached the level of incomplete, with a score of 23 (range, 16 to 23). Performance of the other five functions had also moved upward in quality.

In this agency, the findings of the first audit were distressing to the audit committee, the director, and the staff. The agency was well supported by the community; patients and families often expressed appreciation for nursing service; and there was strong support from the physicians who used the service for their patients. As indicated by the actions reported here, the agency's commitment to quality care quickly transcended its grief at the finding that the overall quality of care could not be rated as good. The distress was increasingly relieved by action that produced measurable results.

In a nursing home certified as an extended care facility, it was decided that all discharged cases would be audited. The first audit of 20 cases showed that the service rendered to patients was of poor quality, with an overall score of 60.8 (range, 41 to 80).

The function of reporting and recording was judged to be at the unsafe level; all other functions, except patient supervision and execution of nursing procedure and techniques, were rated as poor. Execution of both of these two functions was rated as incomplete in quality.

The audit committee recommended increased attention to the recording and reporting function, because it was at the unsafe level,

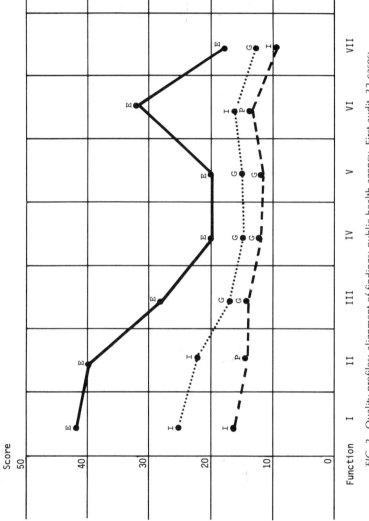

FIG. 2. Quality profiles: alignment of findings; public health agency. First audit, 32 cases; audit 6 months later, 32 cases; and comparison with profile of excellence. Excellence ——————, First Audit – – – –, Audit 6 months later . . . . . . , E Excellent, G Good, I Incomplete, P Poor, U Unsafe.

and to the supervision of patients. The deficits of supervision lay in an almost complete lack of evidence of attention to emotional needs of the patients and to continuing nursing assessments. The care plans were limited to checklists pertaining exclusively to physical care.

The director of this nursing home was dismayed by the audit findings. She had judged staffing to be adequate to provide good care; therefore, she interpreted deficits in care as primarily the result of administrative failure in leadership.

In this facility registered nurses were on duty around the clock, staff ratio was five practical nurses and one nursing aide to one registered nurse during the day, and twice as many practical nurses and nursing aides under the leadership of each registered nurse during the evening and night shifts.

The first change made was in policies in the recording of care. The checklist was being used as the daily "nursing notes," and narrative entries were made every three days. Content of these entries reflected the physical status of patients with respect to personal hygiene, and whether they were in bed, up in a chair, or walking. It included statements about the date and time of physician visits.

The new policy required daily nursing narrative entries which included practical nurse impressions of patient affect. Senior practical nurses, as well as the registered nurses, were made responsible for reviewing each day's charting and for seeing the patients to determine whether they concurred with the entries. If so, they countersigned them. If not, they discussed the care of the patient with the staff member who made the entries, to reconcile differing perceptions of the patients and their situations.

This process resulted in discussions about nursing assessment, with special emphasis on data collection. The public health nurse member of the audit committee was asked to serve as a resource for the nursing staff in relation to data collection.

Attention to the functions of recording and reporting and of supervision of the patient resulted in identification and definition of a number of problems, with action on them. The following examples are illustrative.

1. Patients were assumed by the nursing staff to be clinically stabilized until some critical or unusual signs and symptoms were recognized. The director was of the opinion that she had not sufficiently emphasized the need for alertness to small and subtle changes in patients that would, with nursing intervention, yield secondary prevention results. The interests of the nursing staff in sharpening their observations were aroused by the increased discussion

of patient behavior and its possible meanings. There developed friendly competition in making observations, in understanding patients, and in refining staff attitudes. Nurse care plans became nursing-problem centered.

2. Staffing patterns were recognized as task oriented, which allowed only minimum opportunity for staff-patient interaction. Team nursing was developed during the last quarter of the year in which auditing was initiated.

3. Several practical nurses demonstrated leadership abilities. They were given opportunities to orient new staff and to make rounds with physicians. Two of them were added to the audit committee, which already had one practical nurse.

4. The registered nurses had been spending little time with any but the sickest patients, but much time on managerial tasks. As a group, encouraged by the director, they examined and revised the institutional policy and procedures guides with the help of a nursing consultant from a large local hospital. During this process, it was recognized that some tasks previously considered managerial, but which required nurse performance, could be delegated to nonnursing staff. Other tasks were decided to be unnecessary.

5. Relationships with physicians were altered when nurses began to make rounds with them, discussing patients' potentials as well as present needs. Physicians were asked to write medical notes on the charts each time they saw patients. Later, a review of the notes resulted in medical reexamination and revision of medical policies.

Six months later, the audit showed that overall quality of care had risen to the quality level of incomplete, with a score of 90.4 (range, 81 to 120).

Recording and reporting had risen from the unsafe level to the incomplete level, with a score range of 8 (range, 8 to 11). Supervision of patients was still judged incomplete. But with a score of 14 (range, 10 to 15), this was a four point gain. Improvement of quality in the other five nursing functions was also found, as indicated in Figure 3.

Prior to the use of auditing in this nursing home, all but the sickest patients were found to be receiving highly routinized care. These sickest patients either died or were transferred to acute general hospitals.

Certification and use of the home as an extended care facility were judged by the director to have intensified, but not caused, the focus on tasks and procedures which characterized the nursing service, as revealed in the course of auditing.

When the six-month audit was reviewed with this writer, the di-

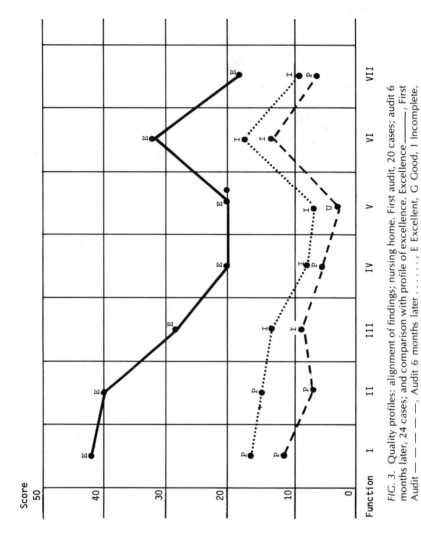

FIG. 3. Quality profiles: alignment of findings; nursing home. First audit, 20 cases; audit 6 months later, 24 cases; and comparison with profile of excellence. Excellence _____, First Audit — — — —, Audit 6 months later . . . . . . , E Excellent, G Good, I Incomplete, P Poor, U Unsafe.

120

rector volunteered that, at the time of the first audit, she had become aware of an unresolved resentment which had affected her leadership. This resentment related to her employment by the nursing home two years earlier. She had, for some years before, administered the nursing service in a large acute general hospital. As a consequence, in her new position, she underestimated the clinical needs of patients and the potentials of a staff less qualified than the one to which she had been accustomed.

One problem that arose as a result of auditing warrants attention. The audit committee recognized from the charts that restraints were sometimes being used on patients at night, without medical orders and in violation of nursing policy. There were nursing notes to the effect that the patients were unruly, uncooperative, and noisy, or aggressive. All these entries were initialed by one nurse. On nights when she was not on duty, there was no record of the use of restraints for these same patients. Nor did these nursing notes reflect problems with the patients.

The committee reported these findings, with the names of patients, verbatim nurses notes, and the dates when restraints were and were not used. After further investigation and validation of events, the nurse was dismissed. This registered nurse had been on staff for 10 years: her performance record throughout the years showed that she was a strong disciplinarian, did not work well with peers, and insisted on working at night "because it was quiet."

While events of this kind do not often occur, auditing in any institution or agency does on occasion reveal serious acts of omission and commission which require administrative action. The audit committee is derelict in its duty if it fails to make full disclosure to the director. It is significant that, in the nursing home situation, the respect for and reliance on the audit committee by the director and the staff were increased by the committee action on the findings which suggested malfeasance.

Auditing reveals problems common to hospitals, public health agencies, and nursing homes that have a bearing on quantity, quality, and costs of care. Nursing appraisals of the physical condition and the observable emotional state of the patient are not ordinarily recorded upon admission or at the time of discharge. Because of this omission, valuable data about the patient are lost, without the possibility of recovering them. Patient behavior at the time of his entry into or discharge from the system of care is particularly revealing, because at those periods he is in transition from a known situation to a new one. His ability, or lack of it, to cope with the change, physically and emotionally, may be more clearly evident at these times than at any other point in his care. The earlier and better the appraisals, the more efficient and effective the care is likely to be.

These nursing appraisals, along with opportunities for guided development by nurses of the skills required to perform them, should be required as a matter of policy.

The planning for continuity of intramural and extramural nursing care leaves much to be desired. Intramurally, nursing summaries and recommendations are not ordinarily made in writing, since the patient moves from one location to another under the same aegis. In each location, therefore, time is lost while nurses essentially begin a new appraisal of the patient in his interactions with the people involved in his care, in his reactions to his condition and causes of illness, and his nursing problems. Policy and procedures which facilitate attention to intramural continuity of care are as important as those which facilitate continuity of care between one type of facility and another.

Assessment of the nursing needs of all patients, selection of the patients who need continuity of care, and the planning for such continuity with them as they move from one setting to another is not yet a general practice.

Referral systems of various types are increasingly used for patients in various clinical or payment categories; yet auditing shows that many patients who have clearly documented needs for continuing nursing care do not receive it.

There appear to be several reasons for this. Referral systems seem basically to be viewed as ends in themselves rather than as a means to continuing care. The mechanism gets more attention than the rationale behind it. The work involved in transmitting information by writing, via whatever referral or transfer form is used, may loom so large through overemphasis as to preclude use of the system in any but the most obvious of cases

The reason most often given by nurses for not planning continuation nursing care is that physicians, who have medical responsibility, often do not agree with the need for continuity of nursing care, and therefore do not order or permit it. One question here is whether the nursing judgment of nursing need is presented forthrightly to the physician, with supporting data on the chart. If this is done, most physicians will consider continuation nursing care for their patients. If the physician will not consider it, the record of the nursing judgment and supporting data remain as evidence that nursing responsibility in supervision of the patient was executed and reported to the physician, to the maximum of feasibility.

If the written nursing judgment, with supporting data, is not made a matter of record on the chart, however, adverse criticism of the physician for not considering continuity of nursing care merely creates or increases interprofessional difficulties. Such difficulties are unpleasant for the professionals, have an adverse effect on the care of patients, and contribute to a nontherapeutic climate in the institution or agency.

Continuation care planning could be expedited by utilization committees. Utilization committees should permit peer-level participation of physicians, nurses, and social workers. The focus should be enlarged from concern with the discharge of patients from a given facility because they no longer need the service therein given, to parallel concern for judgment about what type of continuation care, if any, is specifically required.

In continuation care planning and utilization review, nursing audits provide a hard data base for nursing judgments of the quality of nursing care. These judgments should be brought to bear upon utilization review decisions; all possible economies in the use of health care resources should be attained, but attained without jeopardizing quality of care received by patients.

One major impact of the audit is the resulting institutional or agency profiles of quality that it yields. This emphasis on assessing the quality of care provided to the total population is particularly important in nursing. Nursing practice reflects concern for the general health of all patients. Nursing services are responsible for the impact of nursing on all patients. The nursing process should be meticulously and equally applied in behalf of all patients.

The profiles are particularly important as nursing moves with increasing sophistication to develop appraisals of the outcomes of care, which are essential, and usually and at best center on the results of care for patients with specific diseases. For example, if total populations are not kept in mind, continuation care will be planned for patients with diabetes mellitus, carcinomas, or cardiovascular conditions of an immediately serious nature, but will not be in the lexicon where other patients who need it are involved. Home health services will continue to be thought of as a resource for the aged and chronically ill, but not as a resource for other patients whose health potentials might be realized through use of these services. And preventive and health promoting care that is part of the model of nursing practice will remain in its present, generally embryonic, form.

Perhaps more important in the long run for emphasizing the importance of the total population profile as a part of quality assurance systems is the help it gives in emphasizing disorder instead of disease, that is, in thinking of disease as a process occurring in patients' life spans and life situations. Physician recognition of the need for such help is increasingly evident in medical literature, as illustrated in the following passages:

> We have to think of disorder and not disease, of becoming and not be-ing, of disease as a process and not as an entity. In this way, the physician, himself not long ago a morphologic reductionist, can adapt the concepts of molecular biology to overthrow the physical-chemical atomism so long criticized by him. He has only to remember that disorders occur in persons and that a patient does not carry around a disease as he might a sack of potatoes.[1]

As has been said, the nursing audit is properly to be viewed as one method that fits into the larger context of a quality assurance system. The fit is illustrated by the following experience in one community hospital.

> This hospital has 180 beds and a large ambulatory health care service. Use of the nursing audit was initiated in 1972, after appointment and orientation of the Audit Committee. Experience with the audit led to a system that now includes:
> Peer review of practitioner performance through use of the Slater Nursing Competencies Rating Scale.
> Peer review of the quality of patient care through use of the nursing audit.
> Patients' evaluations of the care they receive are obtained through use of a patient care questionnaire.
> Environmental appraisal through use of a Unit Evaluation check list.
> A Quality Control Committee responsible to the Assistant Administrator of Nursing Services for administration of the Quality Control Program.
> Staff Development Department use of the Quality Control findings in orientation and continuing education of nursing staff and workers responsible to nursing. Staff Development Department efforts are in turn reflected in quality control findings.
> Use of nursing experience in quality assurance to assist in work toward the hospital's over-all goals in quality assurance.[2]

## References

1. Spiro HM: The Tools of the Trade. N Engl J Med 292(11)579, March 13, 1975
2. Sain TR: Nursing Care: Quality Assurance. Detroit, Michigan, Metropolitan Hospital and Health Centers, in press

# Chapter 12
# UNIVERSITY HOSPITAL: NURSING AUDIT EXPERIENCE

Ruth J. Husung, R.N., M.A.,

Nursing audit experience began in University Hospital at the University of Michigan in Ann Arbor during the fall of 1971. In a discussion of the nursing membership on various hospital committees, and as a part of the five-year program for the department, Ann Vose, Director of Nursing, suggested the formation of a nursing audit committee. It was also her request that this writer become chairman of the new committee, which she did, as part of her functions as Coordinator of Departmental Relations.

Thus began a most exciting, satisfying, and rewarding experience for the many nurses who were gradually to join the committee.

This idea of initiating the audit was like planting a little seed which would grow well beyond our expectations.

This chapter reflects the experiences of that growth over a four-year period and looks into the future of the nursing audit.

Once the administrative decisions had been made, the new chairman began her work. A search of the literature in the nearby medical-nursing library uncovered a few references relevant to nursing audit. One item in particular announced that a new book, *The Nursing Audit: Profile for Excellence*, by Maria C. Phaneuf, would be published in 1972. It was to be a guide for nurses who wanted to use the audit regularly as one way of quality control. This book would well serve the purpose of the committee in their beginning efforts to review nursing care in our setting. Thus the search was ended, and efforts were made to obtain the book as soon as possible.

Meanwhile, nurse colleagues located articles already published by Phaneuf and offered suggestions on how to proceed. Incidentally, they also displayed quite an interest in the new venture.

In order to promote and capitalize on such interest, to apprise the nursing staff of the development of the committee, and just possibly recruit members, the chairman outlined plans. These plans were then discussed in prescheduled meetings with head nurse groups and other nursing personnel. They were informed of the plan for establishing an audit committee and doing audits of closed charts, as well as the fact that the director of nursing and the hospital administrators endorsed and would continue support of such efforts. The definition, purpose, methodology, type of membership needed, time constraints, and expected results of the audit were reviewed. Handouts were given to the staff to enable them to learn more about audit. This effort cultivated the "little audit seed," as evidenced by the interest, motivation, knowledge, and hard work which took firm root in our staff.

Shortly thereafter, two staff development instructors volunteered as the first committee members. Thus, the committee began. In meetings which followed, a goal was established to utilize the audit to ascertain the level of nursing care being given in our hospital setting. Word-of-mouth reports indicated that care was good or not so good, depending on who might say it and when. Here, then, was an opportunity to collect data which, hopefully, would help determine what the quality of nursing care was and how to improve it.

The two committee members agreed to serve as a nucleus for the nursing audit and to limit their activities to internal audits. Other members were to include representation from various clinical areas, and the chairman of the audit committee was to be responsible for recruitment. The effort was to be made through the clinical nursing directors and the head nurses, with emphasis on staff nurse participation.

Qualifications for membership included previous audit experience, interest in the plans, willingness to participate, a time commitment to the work, demonstrated ability to work with others, and, most importantly, a modicum of clinical expertise.

When Phaneuf's book was available, a copy was passed along for reading among the committee. Interest centered on the validated schedule which was included in the book, but with no copyright restrictions. Such freedom allowed unlimited reproduction for auditing. This feature, plus all other content, was truly an asset for beginners in the almost overwhelming task of evaluating the quality of nursing care in a large university hospital. Copies of the book were later supplied as a prime reference for each committee member.

Currently, there were five auditors anxious to commence. Since their backgrounds were primarily in medical and surgical nursing, they chose to start with such cases and phase into other areas. So pediatric, maternal and child, psychiatric, and out-patient reviews were deliberately postponed.

Each member reviewed two charts for recently discharged patients in a trial run of auditing. Charts were obtained from patient units according to the auditors' choice. Results were discussed, more trial efforts made, and the members decided that the tool needed to be scrutinized. Soon they ascertained that there must be overlap and duplicate subcomponents which should be eliminated.

Another audit was completed with a revised form, but with everyone evaluating the same chart. Then the members learned a hard lesson: Deletion or revision of any subcomponent necessitates a score revision, which in turn destroys the validity of the tool. Therefore the tool was accepted as published, to be used in our setting.

Other problems confronted the group. Lists of discharges were hard to obtain, retrieval of large numbers of charts was a problem, and then since the auditors were concerned with security and confidentiality of the records in use, the area assigned in which to audit was inadequate. Charts obtained were sometimes mixed, federal funds which paid for the clerk to obtain charts were cut back, and there was no secretary. Delays resulted and auditors had time to wonder if they would even have time for the work. The committee was discouraged, destruction seemed imminent, and the committee questioned whether to even continue with its plans.

Soon the problems were resolved. The books arrived, a secretary was hired, wages became available, adequate space was provided, and medical record staffing improved as did the service. Without such support, the audit would have been doomed.

A year passed and recruitment of new members started, as is usual after that length of time. As nurses heard about auditing, some volunteered. For example, a recent experience is evidence of a trend. During an orientation class for recently employed nurses, information about the audit committee functions and achievements was presented. Anyone interested in becoming a member was invited to stop by after class. Out of a class of 40, ten signed up for the committee. Recruitment is a selling job, and such results are gratifying. A volunteer is highly motivated and truly an asset.

To date about 50 people, including two licensed practical nurses, have shared in and contributed to the audit experience. Membership has varied from new graduates to faculty members with much nursing experience. All the nurses had been women until recently, when one male nurse joined the committee.

The length of time a committee member stays with the group has varied from a few months to a couple of years. There always has been at least one nurse from each of the seven clinical areas in this hospital, as the areas were included in the audit. Audit time has generally been on duty hours, with overtime pay allowed, if there was no other way to manage. Though often reluctant because of the interest and satisfaction they found in the work, members leave the group in order to allow others the opportunity to be involved.

The orientation of members is of great importance to success in auditing. Initially, an overview of the work is given, along with an explanation of the purpose and methodology. The concept that documentation is an important part of nursing care, and that it reflects or mirrors actual provision of care must be accepted. So far, only one nurse recruit could not endorse the ideas, admitted to her disbelief, and did not remain with the group.

Because of information contained in patient records, confidentiality has been constantly stressed by the chairman. It helps to protect the rights of patients and to help keep the standards high for the committee. High levels of performance by the auditors lends credence to their efforts as they evaluate nursing care given by their peers. Punitive attitudes toward individuals rendering poor care are thus prevented. Forgetting names on charts is likewise fostered.

In orientation, a recruit generally does one audit for practice, and results are reviewed with the chairman or the member whom she is replacing. Audit results are compared with the actual audit done by a regular member. The steps are repeated, and the recruit may pace herself to gradually begin to review two or three charts officially. Thus skill is developed, and confidence gained. Assistance is nearby as requested or needed by the recruit.

For variation in their orientation, new members have met together with the chairman in miniworkshops to audit a chart together. This approach is repeated once. Charts copied for these sessions have been chosen for cases having 10- to 14-day hospital stays and of particular clinical interest to the group.

The next step is to expand auditing to the usual 7 to 10 charts, which has been an average number for each auditor every month. Usually, three weeks have been allowed for completion of the monthly quota. It has often been a pleasant surprise for the newer member to realize how readily skill is developed and the ease with which important judgments about quality can be made. One other little surprise has been to note that to audit well is to think, and how much like giving good care this is.

About every three months, the committee reviews a copy of the same chart together in a meeting. Components are discussed, definitions used, and consensus reached. Interrater reliability is thus affirmed, and new members are aided in learning. These efforts are a source of satisfaction and edification for everyone.

Occasionally, for variety, each person has individually audited the same chart prior to a meeting where results were discussed. Great discourses have ensued, and group dynamics have propelled the members forward. The exchanges are fruitful.

Members early defined a need for regularly scheduled meetings, so the third Wednesday of each month was set up and maintained, and no meeting has ever been cancelled. Attendance has never been mandatory, yet an element of responsibility and an appreciation of membership on the committee has been evident when the members attend even during days off.

In most of the meetings, data from audits are discussed. The excellent and poor cases are given special study to ascertain the significance of the findings. Recommendations have been made on the basis of the data.

A planned agenda fosters freedom of discussion, communication, flexibility, and a sense of progress and accomplishment necessary for a viable, working relationship.

Membership has grown to a recent all-time high of 20. Currently, there are 16 auditors, with some ready to phase out, while about 15 staff nurses are waiting to join.

After six months of auditing was finished, the committee was well established. There were enough new members to expand the audit to the entire hospital except for the out-patient area, rather than to phase in areas as had been planned initially.

Commendations of work well done had come from the nursing and hospital directors. Colleagues were congratulating the committee. This encouraged them to expand their efforts.

As indicated previously, as soon as the auditors were ready for regular, systematic work, selection of charts was necessary. A randomized sample was chosen from a monthly, computer printout of patient names and registration numbers. An average of 2000 discharges occur each month. Because of the small size of the committee, especially at the beginning, a mutual decision was made to select 5 percent of the charts, rather than the 10 percent suggested in the book.

To audit, each member removes a chart from the top of a box marked with the registration numbers for that batch and signs off the chart on a list provided. Once reviewed, the chart goes back to a file area and thus leaves the audit review. Completed audits have always been placed in a designated envelope. These steps serve to prevent replication of a completed audit, and any possible identification on the chart that an audit has been done. To do otherwise might lead to misuse of evidence, if care were less than good and might violate the confidence entrusted to each auditor.

Each patient record is reviewed only by one auditor. Care is taken, if patients have had multiple admissions, to audit the section for the month being evaluated. If, by chance, there was more than one admission in the time period, the longer interval is audited. Scoring has been done by the secretary, although the members have practiced, so they can teach the technique in workshops in which they may participate.

An interesting omission of answers occurs periodically. No particular patterns have been seen, and reminders tend to reduce them. The auditors need to be shaped up with a measure of discipline once in awhile.

Written remarks have been encouraged on every audit and are later summarized for the month by members who volunteer to do it. Comments have been both negative and positive relative to the findings in the review of the chart and have supported the data.

The assistance of a secretary to provide the usual support services has been essential to the committee function. From the start, the job has been filled by a student nurse. The clinical background of the student has facilitated the work, and freed the nurse auditors for the actual audit with the critical decision making.

Several students have held the secretarial job, and each has been amazed at the knowledge and insight gained about nursing care, as they go through charts in order to fill in the front of the audit tool. Needless to say, having a student nurse is cost effective compared with the higher wages of regular secretaries or nurses.

Ever mindful of costs of health care, the auditors learn early to discipline themselves to complete an audit in a minimum of time (never to exceed two hours), and yet be thorough and just in the evaluation. They are encouraged to scan the chart and to avoid the inevitable human tendency to read more because "it is so interesting." Costs are essentially for time spent for audit, materials, books and salary for the secretary. An annual budget has been around $15,000, a small sum to help assure quality of care.

After the first month of auditing, the first audit report was written and forwarded to the director of nursing. There were four parts to the report: (1) statistical summary and quality profile, (2) summary of basic identifying data, (3) remarks written by the audit committee, (4) recommendation(s) from the committee. The format has stayed the same except for the addition of part 5, summary of recommendation(s) to date, as more reports were generated. Distribution of reports has expanded from the clinical nursing directors to include all head nurses and staff, medical staff quality assurance committee members, charting committee, hospital administrators, staff development instructors, university school of nursing faculty, and all others interested.

During the past year, an exciting breakthrough occurred when the data systems staff became interested in the nursing audit tool, and put it on computer as a teaching aid for their staff. Eventually, the audit tool was put on computer and later programmed for audit data input with a production file. The last two audit reports have been compiled utilizing the computer printouts. This has been a breakthrough for the secretary and the auditors, for the time and effort saved is used for more careful review of data and greater in-depth evaluations.

To date, approximately 1800 records have been audited by nurses. A total of 19 reports have been written for the monthly audits, and several more have been written for special audits done at the request of staff for their unit.

Time lags have occurred in these developments, fluctuating with staff shortages, high census, vacations, committee and secretary turnover, and delays in obtaining charts regularly. To cope with the lapse of time, to be closer to real time with audits, only a six-month period is audited. The cycle has been June through November. One batch was completed for February 1974, to see if a winter month might show different data. Essentially, it did not. The six-month rotation has been well accepted too for the ease of comparing each succeeding year.

Every report has included the overall evaluation by number of cases. Table 1 shows this information in totals for June through November during the past three years. It is evident that by 1974, more cases were in the good and excellent categories, which indicates improvement in care given.

Very early in auditing, the committee theorized that the length of

**TABLE 1**
**Overall Evaluation by Number of Cases**
**Medical-Surgical, 1972, All Cases, 1973 to 1974**

| Year | Excel- lent | Good | Incom- plete | Poor | Unaccept- able | Total |
|---|---|---|---|---|---|---|
| 1972 | 23 | 109 | 139 | 79 | 8 | 358 |
| 1973 | 102 | 278 | 190 | 72 | 9 | 648 |
| 1974 | 153 | 250 | 134 | 29 | 6 | 581 |
| Total | 278 | 637 | 463 | 180 | 23 | 1587 |

stay for patients might influence the care, for example short stay, poor care; long stay, good care. The range of days for the admission was figured for each case. Findings have continually indicated that the quality of care has ranged from unacceptable to excellent, irrespective of the length of stay.

With the finalization of three years of auditing, comparison of data was urgently desired. At one time earlier, the staff in the medical record department had offered to assist the audit committee in such compilations. And thus they became involved in helping with the summations included in this chapter.

Figure 1 shows the overall scores for the monthly audits done over a three-year period. Obviously, steady overall improvement is evident, as reflected in the increase of the scores.

Each month as the audit scores were tallied, there was great anticipation to learn what the quality profile would be. Each such profile has been compared with the Profile for Excellence in *The Nursing Audit*. The first profile for University Hospital showed that the care was incomplete in some areas and good in others. However, that result was typical in such settings, and recommendations were made for improvement. In each succeeding year of audit, there has been a noteworthy improvement in all nursing functions evaluated except the seventh, as shown in Figure 2. An elaboration on the progress seems appropriate.

Function I, application and execution of physician's legal orders, was good. In the past two years, this dependent function has become excellent, which simply means that nurses have carried out the components of care quite well.

Function II, observation of symptoms and reactions, was in the good range each year and was almost excellent in 1974. Good knowledge about diseases, therapy, and the patient's position related to his disease or illness have been evidenced by the nursing staff.

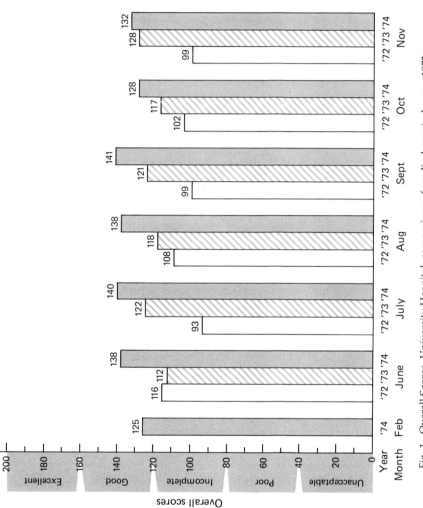

*Fig. 1.* Overall Scores, University Hospital, comparison of medical-surgical cases, 1972; all cases June through November, 1973 and 1974, and February, 1974.

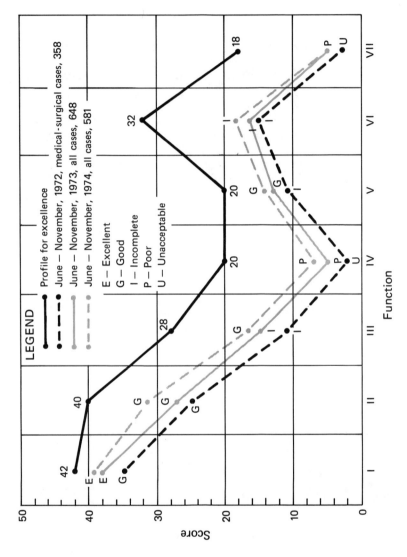

LEGEND

| | |
|---|---|
| ——— | Profile for excellence |
| ● – – – ● | June – November, 1972, medical-surgical cases, 358 |
| ● ——— ● | June – November, 1973, all cases, 648 |
| ● – – – ● | June – November, 1974, all cases, 581 |

E – Excellent
G – Good
I – Incomplete
P – Poor
U – Unacceptable

*Fig. 2.* Quality profiles: alignment of findings, University Hospital.

Function III, supervision of the patient, was in the incomplete range until the past year, when it improved to the good range. Lack of follow-up with all assessments and slow development of nursing diagnoses may account for delay.

Function IV, supervision of those participating in care (except the physician), has been slowly moving from the lower ranges. Evidence shows that the teaching and emotional components for patients and families, however, is good sometimes, but could be better.

Function V, reporting and recording, was almost good, then moved into that range and stayed there. The advocacy of improved documentation for the facts established by staff in relation to the patient's condition, and primary disease, has brought some improvement.

Function VI, application and execution of nursing procedures and techniques, has remained incomplete. The committee feels that the performance of this function will continue to move upward. The old attitude which negated the importance of performing this function has gradually changed.

Function VII, promotion of physical and emotional health by direction and teaching, has been slow to move upward and then has stayed the same for two years. Many staff members hold the belief that in this teaching hospital, instruction is given to patients and families but has not generally been recorded by nurses. New policies which stress more planning for the discharge of the patient prior to leaving the hospital, and summation of nursing care given, should help improve this function.

The reports indicate further that no regression in any of the nursing functions has taken place. This overall, general progression in improvement toward excellence in the nursing care functions described has been encouraging.

In basic identifying data, the greatest change has been in the increased number of complete signatures and titles of nursing staff who make notes on the patient records. Systems charting, and even better handwriting, have increased the references by the physicians and other nursing staff to the nurses' documentation, and facilitates auditing.

Finally, in each audit report are the recommendations made by the committee based on audit data. They are made in a meeting where the findings have been reviewed. From one to four have been developed each time. There has been some repetition of the recommendations, but with emphasis on subcomponents. Thus far 35 recommendations have been made with an emphasis on their implementation to improve care.

In the first audits, documentation was limited, thus the first recommendation encouraged formation of a charting committee to set up standards and improve the forms for nursing records. Other recommendations have stressed the need to improve all seven nursing functions, in order to provide a holistic approach to care and personalization of that care for each patient, to the best level possible. Patient assessments have needed more follow-up.

Other recommendations have encouraged staff to be more aware of reactions by patients, to include the patient and family more in care and planning, and to better instruct them in what and when to report to the physician.

Finally, even greater attention than in the past has been advised for the patient's comfort and emotional support, and summaries of teaching and planning for the patient's discharge.

As soon as the reports were completed, they were distributed with the intent that they be shared with staff and implemented. The clinical nursing directors and head nurses share in such responsibilities and are to be commended for their constant support and tireless efforts for the improvement of patient care.

Various efforts have been made to assist and encourage staff to take action on the findings of the audit, to build on the strengths, and eliminate the weaknesses. Miniworkshops and progress reports on audit have been given by committee members to the head nurses and other staff. Presentation of the purpose and methodology of auditing, along with copies of the recommendations, have been presented during orientation for new nursing staff. The use of the 50 subcomponents in the audit tool have been suggested as a guide to planning, giving, and recording nursing care.

The example set by committee members themselves effectively involve nurses in use of the audit findings. As each auditor has learned about the effect audit findings can have to improve care, efforts have increased to quietly practice what is preached. A nursing newsletter with wide distribution in the hospital carries progress notes about auditing. Thus the audit findings branch out, care is better—a patient rests peacefully.

Possibilities of phasing in some type of audit in the outpatient clinical areas continue to be explored. Similar examinations and discussions have stimulated emergency room staff to conduct reviews for a sample of patients admitted from there to special care and other units. Findings have helped the nurses better define their role and the need for new forms on which to record care.

Several special audits have been done. More have been requested and will be done with the help of computer reports. One of the special audits is noteworthy as an indication of trends. The medical staff has been cognizant of the nursing audit. After completion of one of their own audits, medical staff shared the results with nursing, and then the nurse auditors consented to review the same batch of 25 charts. The cases had been chosen because the patients had been admitted to intensive care. Audit findings were exciting, for nursing care was excellent. The nurses attributed the high level of care to the fact that the ratio of staff was high for each patient. The evidence underscored the effects of good staffing. The audit was the first of its kind used in collaboration with physicians for the evaluation of patient care.

A few spin-offs have come rather unexpectedly from the audit to enhance the experience. Other departments within the hospital have asked for input from the committee about the activity. Invitations to participate in workshops on audit in the state, and elsewhere, have been accepted by the auditors. Lastly, some proceedings of the audit committee were featured in an article, "Nursing audit: New yardstick for patient care," written by Charlotte Isler.*

Presently, the nursing audit experience continues to grow. The time lag is being reduced as auditors finish the review of records for patients discharged in June 1975. Thus, another cycle of six months of systematic, retrospective audit begins. Computer input of audit data continues with a new student nurse as secretary. New lists for audits are compiled. New members prepare for a new experience, to audit. More reports with recommendations will be distributed for implementation. A great audit tree from a tiny audit seed grows!

A quality assurance program is developing well, within the department of nursing, including evaluation of outcomes of care. Plans for the future include a continuation of the nursing audit committee for review and evaluation of the nursing process, as an integral part of the nursing quality assurance program. With such self-regulation, nurses will be accountable for the care given to patients and for the results of the care.

In summary, a retrospective review of the nursing audit experience at University Hospital reflects continuous development of committee membership and efforts to implement the audit findings. Progressive movement of the seven nursing functions toward Phaneuf's profile for excellence has shown an overall improvement in nursing care. The quality of the care given is judged to be good.

*RN 37(12):31, December 1974.

The outcomes of these interrelated, dynamic efforts are indicators of more experience of the kind reflected in this chapter. Based on audit findings, and future plans, the assurance of quality care for future patients at University Hospital is concurrently evident.

# Chapter 13
# VISITING NURSE AGENCY: NURSING AUDIT EXPERIENCE

Sylvia R. Peabody, R.N., M.S.N.

The administration of a nursing service requires the acceptance of responsibility for accountability to the public for the quality of the service delivered. Agencies such as The Visiting Nurse Association (VNA) of Metropolitan Detroit have traditionally reported to the public regularly on their services through their Board of Trustees, annual meetings, brochures, and publicity. They have assumed that if the structure meets high standards, the quality of service will be good. This is the rationale for the National League for Nursing's Program of Accreditation of Home Health Agencies and Community Nursing Services. Although this peer review of structure is one step in the assessment of the quality of nursing service, it does not really look at the actual nursing service delivered. The examination of nursing process as the care is being delivered or retrospectively on completed service could provide better information on the quality of service. The third method, the study of the results of service—outcomes is not easy, since many other factors besides nursing, such as medical care and family support, are difficult to control or rule out as factors in the outcome. The Phaneuf Nursing Audit was already available and seemed to be the one instrument which was practical and could be used immediately to examine retrospectively the quality of nursing service delivered. The staff recommended this to the Board of Trustees, and it was approved for implementation in the summer of 1970. The nursing audit has been an ongoing program of the Detroit VNA ever since, with regular audits nine times a year.

The VNA of Metropolitan Detroit serves most of a three county area of over 1200 square miles and has eight district offices and three neighborhood clinics. Over 300 persons comprise its multidisciplinary staff with nurses, therapists, social workers, nutritionists, nurse clinicians, and consultants in maternity, pediatrics, and mental health. This variety provides a richness of resources for patient and family service. The decentralization of staff is essential for economy of travel and also to have manageable staff groupings for in-service education, district management, and supervision. However, with the advantages, there are concomitant problems, including varied methods of policy implementation, special interests of supervisors, varying leadership styles, and some inconsistencies in monitoring of case management, in guidance of staff in the development and refinement of skills, and use of the nursing process. The institution of the nursing audit seemed to lend itself to identifying problem areas in the delivery of service and in interpretation and implementation of agency policies which affect the quality of care.

In July and August of 1970, a public health nursing faculty member from Wayne State University was employed full time as audit consultant to introduce the nursing audit to all staff, train the audit committee, and in general, to help the VNA get a good start in all aspects of the audit.

The first phase was initial orientation of all staff. It took about a month to hold conferences and discussions in each district office about the audit's purpose, goals for this agency, limitations, and possible outcomes. Some staff members were quite verbal and defensive about any implied criticism of service and recording. For the most part, however, there was general interest and a recognition of the need for accountability. The audit guide and audit review procedures were reviewed with emphasis on the seven nursing functions which were to be assessed. A sample of an audited record was reviewed and discussed. Some of the kinds of questions raised by staff included how the audit could result in improved in-service education, the problem of time spent in recording service more completely, and how staff can learn about recommendations made by the audit committee.

The audit committee was appointed and consisted of eight representatives of district offices (five field staff and three supervisors), one administrator (and alternate), one nurse (and alternate) from a nearby hospital (which was also introducing the nursing audit). Later, when a VNA consultant in medical-surgical nursing was employed, the responsibility of staffing the audit committee was assigned to her.

The second phase of introduction of the nursing audit was the training of the audit committee, the development of an agency philosophy and objectives for the ongoing use of the audit, and policies on how to handle findings of the audits.

The audit consultant selected a VNA record which had several problems typical of those the committee would be dealing with regularly, such as missing information, temptation to assume nursing actions which were not documented, etc. The committee used the record to go through each step of the audit and to develop an acceptable way of coping with the problems as they occurred. When the scoring was completed, the committee analyzed the results and identified the strengths and weaknesses in the quality of care. They discussed what to do with findings and recognized that as a group of records are audited, the frequency of weakness in an area will indicate some needed action. This would be the kind of problem to be identified to the executive director with recommendations for action.

Several members of the audit committee worked as a subcommittee in drafting a statement of philosophy, beliefs about patients' rights, beliefs about nursing actions, and objectives for the audit committee. Since the philosophy and beliefs were quite global and later were refined and developed into an agency philosophy, they are not included here, but the objectives of the audit committee are pertinent:

The overall objective of the audit committee is to improve the quality of nursing care. The contributory objectives are the following:

1. To identify strengths and weaknesses in nursing care provided to patients and families
2. To determine whether the agency record reflects the quality of care given
3. To identify problems which interfere with the giving of quality nursing care to patients and families
4. To report all findings and make recommendations to the executive director for improvement in the quality of nursing care
5. To assess whether improved quality of service does result from changes instigated as a result of the audit committee's recommendations

The third phase in the institution of the audit in the VNA was practice in auditing a group of records independently. The committee decided what types of cases to select, and the records were obtained from several district offices. The records were audited independently and then discussed. Differences in judgment on scoring and in interpretation of definitions were resolved. The results of the practice audit on this group of records were analyzed, and the beginning recognition of common weaknesses in service given emerged. Several recommendations were formulated for future consideration if the results of auditing a larger group of records validated these same weaknesses.

The committee prepared for the last phase—a trial run on a 10 percent sample of discharged patients' records, excluding maternal and child health. They discussed ways of developing skill and speed in auditing through practice, a quiet place for concentration away from their own offices, preparatory work, and tabulation by a trained clerk. Since case and family records are not centralized and are not numbered in a way that could be used with random numbers for selecting records for audit, another scheme was devised. Security for records was established, they were to be transported in special expandable files. Each audit committee member would be assigned the records from one or two district offices other than her own. She was to plan her own time for auditing her assigned records. Her scored audit sheets were to be turned in to the clerk for tabulation. The committee was ready to proceed with the trial run.

The trial run was highly successful—the last phase began. The 10 percent sample produced 74 closed records which were audited. The committee members were diligent in their work. They were also surprised that more than half were Incomplete, Poor, or Unsafe in the nursing care recorded. The committee analyzed the areas of strength and weakness and made the following recommendations to the executive director:

1. Each RN should have a manometer and stethoscope with some additional ones in the office available for LPNs to use.
2. Record policies need to be reinforced and amended to require the nurse's signature (instead of initials) and professional title (R.N., L.P.N., etc.).
3. Supervisors should make recording the subject of an in-service education program in each district to review *Guide to the Use of the Service Record.*
4. All medical orders on the record should show name and title of person transcribing orders, as well as date received, name of physician, address, and telephone number.

All these recommendations were of great concern to the committee. Each district received the scores for that district and for the VNA as a whole. Some had no Poor or Unsafe scores, and it was easy to note where the most work needed to be done either on recording or on quality of care. At this early stage, the nurses tended to believe that recording was the greater problem. They were reminded by their audit committee member that the audit motto had become "if it's not recorded, it wasn't done."

The Phaneuf Nursing Audit is very adaptable to whatever needs study. Over the years, we have audited maternal and child health service; diagnostic categories, such as patients with diabetes, heart and circulatory problems, neurologic problems, malignancies, orthopedic problems, lung pathology, strokes; and other interests, like the nurse's use of consultants, service to various age groups—especially the aged and pediatrics. The audit committee selects the kind of records to be audited the next month, and sometimes for a series of months. The variety of nursing audits which have been done have given a new stimulus to staff and their supervisors to improve their nursing practice and the way it is recorded.

We are very gratified that the audits have shown great improvement since that first trial run. Although there are still one or two Unsafe records in most audits, there are 75 percent to 85 percent which are Good or Excellent. The minutes of the committee show their own concern about areas which are consistently low, even though the total record score is good.

Orientation to the nursing audit is held annually, and the districts appoint new representatives so that more staff get a deep exposure to the process, the concerns, and what needs to be done to improve nursing service. We believe this kind of involvement has made a significant difference in the acceptance of the findings and the desire to improve the quality of nursing delivered by this VNA.

The benefits growing out of the use of the nursing audit are numerous. Some of the most significant are the following:

1. The development of an agency philosophy and objectives for each service
2. The ongoing work of developing nursing actions to accomplish objectives in service to patients with cancer, diabetes, stroke, and lung pathology
3. Improved equipment and skills for nursing assessment and diagnosis
4. Increased in-service education related to problems identified in the audit
5. Employment of nurse clinicians in adult health, mental health, and pediatrics to give direct clinical service and to guide staff through consultation, shared visits, and in-service education
6. Plans for full implementation of a problem-oriented record system
7. The development of a patient information system which includes outcome measures which we hope can be correlated with nursing audit results

Since the introduction of the nursing audit to this VNA in 1970, great progress has been made in the acceptance by staff at all levels for accountability to consumers for the quality of service provided. We are planning the development of a system of quality assurance for this agency which includes the nursing audit and which could be a model for other agencies. The future power of governmental regulations including the health systems agencies and PSROs can be appropriately controlled for nursing service, if the nursing profession can develop models of quality assurance in which government, third parties, and the medical profession can have confidence. We believe nursing can and must retain control of nursing practice.

# Chapter 14

# THE SLATER NURSING COMPETENCIES RATING SCALE AND THE QUALITY PATIENT CARE SCALE

## Mabel A. Wandelt R.N., Ph.D.

The Slater Nursing Competencies Rating Scale and the Quality Patient Care Scale are two more instruments for measuring the quality of the process component of nursing care. Each shares in common with the audit several important attributes:

They provide reliable and relevant quantitative and descriptive measurements of a comprehensive gamut of nursing care actions composing the process of nursing care for patients.

They are designed to measure the quality of nursing care provided in any setting where nurse-patient interactions occur.

The standard of measurement for each is held constant. This is an attribute different from most tools developed for measuring nursing performance or nursing care. Most other tools use sliding scales that go into great descriptions about ways to rate observed performance or care in terms of what you expect of the individual performing the care or for the patient receiving the care. The sliding scale does not work, because it provides no means for comparing one with another. The audit and the two scales each utilize a standard of measurement held constant regardless of whose performance is being measured—a sophomore student, a senior student, a nurse aide, or a nurse clinician—or regardless of characteristics of the patient receiving care—young or old, fully conscious or comatose, suffering fractured femur or lobar pneumonia. The constant standard of measurement is used for rating the various dimensions of care being measured. If, then, there are the differences expected, they will be revealed in the measurements made with either of the scales or the audit instrument.

Quantitative measurements are sufficiently sensitive to identify discriminations where differences in quality exist.

Descriptive measurements are readily identified with components of the nursing practice process and setting from which the measurements were obtained and, therefore, serve for expeditious planning of changes calculated to improve the practice.

In addition to the commonalities, there are differences in the three instruments. The differences are fortunate, since information about quality of nursing care is sought for various purposes, and situations and circumstances in which measurements will be done also vary. In some instances, any of the instruments or all three would serve; in others, one instrument provides advantages over the others. In this chapter, there will be brief descriptions of the scales and their use, followed by some factors to be considered when selecting the instrument to be used for obtaining measurements for particular purposes or in particular situations.

# SLATER NURSING COMPETENCIES RATING SCALE

The Slater Nursing Competencies Rating Scale is an 84-item scale designed to measure the competencies displayed by a nurse as she performs nurse actions in providing care to patients. The Scale may be used in any setting where nurses intervene in behalf of patients, either in direct nurse-patient interactions or in other interventions.

The Scale is used, in retrospect, to rate nurse performance that has occurred over a period of time, anywhere from two weeks to one year, or for on-the-spot ratings. For ratings of performance occurring over a period of time, the rater is a nurse who has observed the subject to be rated as she provided direct nursing care for patients over the duration of the rating period. The rater ascribes ratings to the items on the Scale on the basis of retrospective analysis of the many observations witnessed of episodes of care being provided by the subject during the rating period.

For some purposes, the Scale may be used for ratings during a one-time observation period. For this on-the-spot rating, the nurse observer shadows the nurse to be rated as she provides care for patients during a 2.5-hour period. She ascribes rating to one or more germane items for each episode of the nurse's interactions with or interventions on behalf of patients.

**Table 1**

| Area | Number of items |
|---|---|
| 1. *Psychosocial: Individual.* Actions directed toward meeting psychosocial needs of individual patients | 18 |
| 2. *Psychosocial: Group.* Actions directed toward meeting psychosocial needs of patients as members of a group | 13 |
| 3. *Physical.* Actions directed toward meeting physical needs of patients | 13 |
| 4. *General.* Actions that may be directed toward meeting either psychosocial or physical needs of patient or both at once | 16 |
| 5. *Communication.* Communication on behalf of patient | 7 |
| 6. *Professional Implications.* Care given to patients reflects initiative and responsibility indicative of professional expectations | 17 |
| Total items | 84 |

The 84 items are arranged into six subsections, as outlined in Table 1, according to the primary science and cultural bases for the nursing care actions to be rated.

The items are identified in terms descriptive of observable nurse actions, which enables the term to be readily matched with criterion measures for behaviorally stated objectives of a nursing service or educational program.

Among the purposes for which measurements from the Slater Scale may serve are the following:

Periodic personnel evaluations of individual nurses, where retention, promotion, and merit salary increases are among the considerations

Where administration is interested in examining relationships between competencies displayed by nurses and the quality of care received by patients

To identify areas of needed instruction for in-service educational programs or particular learning needs of individual staff members

Investigations to determine relationships between one or more components of nursing care and the quality of the performance of nursing personnel providing care to patients

Essentially, where there is interest in knowing the level of competency displayed by a nurse, for whatever reason, the Slater Scale will provide a discriminating measurement for each individual or group of individuals measured. The Scale has been repeatedly demonstrated to be so sensitive that it will measure changes that occur (learning) in as brief a time as two weeks.

# QUALITY PATIENT CARE SCALE

The Quality Patient Care Scale (Qualpacs) is a 68-item scale designed to measure the quality of care received by patients in any setting in which nurses intervene to provide care for patients, either in direct nurse-patient interactions or in interventions in behalf of the patient. Qualpacs derived from the Slater Scale. Many of the items from the Slater fit into Qualpacs by merely structuring the wording to describe the nurse action as it was received by the patient, rather than as it was performed by the nurse.

The items are arranged into the same six subsections, and the items are identified in terms descriptive of observable nurse actions.

Ratings of care for a patient are done by a nurse who spends two hours in direct observation of the care provided to the patient. On the basis of observed interactions and of information from the patient's record and from members of the staff, the nurse ascribes ratings to all applicable items on the scale. As for the Slater Scale, the numerical values for the items are ascribed when the total rating for care has been completed.

Greater detail about the Scales can be found in the original articles, and there is full description of their content and use in the individual publication of each.[1,2] For purposes of this presentation, additional comments will be limited to considerations germane to selection of tools to be used for systematic evaluation of quality of nursing care.

Quality assurance is a term with various meanings for various people. Its meanings include provision of evidence of meeting agreed levels of excellence, ie, evidence of maintaining a standard. Implied is an accounting to someone for something one has done or produced. Commonly, when used in reference to health care, it is used in relation to PSRO legislation and physician accountability for the level of quality of care they provide. The accounting involves providing evidence of the level of excellence of the outcome of medical care provided patients, as compared to a standard for the particular locale in which the care is provided. Some view quality assurance in a larger sense; that is, not only as an accounting for the current level of care, but also as a commitment to improvement of the care and professional practice in general. Whether the program be viewed as limited to accounting or, more broadly, as extending to providing for improvement, evaluation is the essence of the program.

Evaluation, as well as quality assurance, is a term having multiple connotations; each is frequently used interchangeably with terms associated with it, and sometimes they are interchanged with each other. Because this is so, it is well to make explicit what is meant as the terms are used in any particular context. It is well to begin by clearly identifying what evaluation is, what measurement is, and what their relationship to each other is. Both measurement and evaluation have two distinct meanings, related to the process of accomplishing each.

Measurement, as a process, is the ascertaining of the dimensions, quantity, or capacity of something, usually by comparing a single phenomenon with a standard of measurement.

Measurement, as a result of the process, is the recorded number or symbol that represents the magnitude of the phenomenon in terms of the magnitude of the standard of measurement.

Evaluation, as a process, is the ascertaining or fixing of the value or worth of a person or thing. The process includes considered judgment.

Evaluation, as a result of the process, is a generalization describing a judgment of the value or worth of a person or thing. An evaluation is a generalization describing a judgment based on many measurements.

It is helpful to think of evaluation as a process of gathering information that may be used to serve various purposes:

1. To account for the level of care provided
2. To make comparisons (of different situations, settings, or times)
   a. To determine the effects of changes made in care practices
   b. To determine differences in care
   c. To determine the extent to which objectives of a program have been attained
3. To provide bases for planning for improvement

These general purposes to be served by information obtained through evaluations apply whether concern is for programs of service, education, or research, or whether for groups or individuals.

The three tools provide measurements of the quality of the process of nursing care provided patients. Each yields two categories of measurements, quantitative and descriptive. Where the purpose for seeking information is to account to someone for the quality of care provided or for making comparisons, the usual and most precise measurements are the quantitative ones.

Where information is sought for the purpose of planning changes in program with the view to improvement, the descriptive data provide the base for planning and decisions.

The quantitative measurements can tell us our level of attainment, they can provide for comparisons of various kinds, and they can serve for accounting for our practice. Thus they can alert us to areas of strength and of weakness, but only the descriptive measurements provide information that guides to planning improvement. It is proposed that the most important purpose to be served by evaluation endeavors is the securing of information that can lead to improvement. If this idea were more readily accepted and more frequently recognized, evaluation might be approached with more positive attitudes. This is particularly so in relation to evaluations of individual performance. If, instead of viewing evaluation as criticism, fault or error identification, and something to be gotten over with and forgotten, it were viewed as means to learning ways to improve oneself, evaluation might become the ongoing process that makes it most effective, and it might be welcomed as an expression of interested, helping concern.

Evaluation endeavors may be limited to periodic episodes, with information used to account for practice only. Or the evaluation may be established as an ongoing program of varying degrees of detail and complexity wherein, along with securing quantitative measurements, descriptive measurements are also recorded with the intent to use the information as a base for improvement of the entities measured.

The preceding background serves as a base for identifying factors to be considered when selecting from among the three tools the one or ones to be used for a particular evaluation project.

## FACTORS TO BE CONSIDERED IN TOOL SELECTION

The measurements obtained with the Slater Scale are those of the quality of the performance of an individual as she provides care for patients. If concern is about the performance of an individual or individuals, whether in relation to continuing employment, changes in assignment, learning in an educational program, or many other elements associated with a person's performance, the Slater Scale would be the tool to be used. The information from the Slater Scale will serve to account for individual or group performance, to identify areas of strengths and weaknesses, and to provide guides to elements of performance needing improvement, for either individuals or groups.

The Nursing Audit and the Qualpacs yield measurements of the quality of care received by patients. Each yields quantitative and descriptive data; general evaluation purposes may be met through the use of either instrument. There are, however, associated factors that may dictate the instrument to be used at a particular time. The initial cost of using the Qualpacs is less than that for using the Nursing Audit. As few as two persons are all that are needed to use the Qualpacs, and it requires only two days for nurses to learn to use the Qualpacs sufficiently well to secure reliable measurements with it. Learning to use the audit requires a considerably longer period of time, and there must be at least five nurses intimately involved. But once the audit committee has become oriented to use of the audit, a monthly evaluation of a total nursing service can be accomplished with expenditure of less than 20 hours of professional nurse time. Whereas, each episode of evaluation with use of the Qualpacs must be calculated in terms of 1.5 to 2 nurse days per nursing unit. Definitive measures can be obtained sooner with Qualpacs; over the long range, the Audit is less costly for repeated measurements, that is, for continual monitoring.

Each tool yields information about strengths and weaknesses. Each tool, through its very use, prompts movement to improve nursing care practices among the nursing staff. The Qualpacs makes those using it aware of subtle components of comprehensive care, and to a limited degree, the users may alert their colleagues. With the Qualpacs, most movement toward improvement follows analysis of the findings from the use of the scale and the planning and formalizing of projects and actions for improving the nursing practice. On the other hand, the Nursing Audit leads the users, even before they have fully learned to audit, to marked improvement in their own practice and to involving and leading all co-workers, head nurse, staff nurse, and nurse aide, to increased awareness of elements of comprehensive care and to improved practice. With the Nursing Audit, there is a marked and noticeable movement toward improvement in care by the time members of the audit committee have audited a dozen records. Because of this phenomenon, all personnel enter more readily into planning and actions for improvements in the nursing care program. Indeed, many initiate or demand improvements before administration has suggested them, or sometimes, even before it is ready to provide them. If decision is to launch an evaluation program with the view to moving into a long-range continuing program, decision may well be to begin with the Nursing Audit.

As mentioned, each tool serves to remind nurses of the many components of comprehensive nursing care. The items of the tools serve to identify specific elements of care that are or are not being provided. Where it is planned that emphasis will be placed on improving practice of registered nurse staff, the Nursing Audit may be the preferred tool. Where the program for improvement will focus on the auxiliary nursing staff, the Qualpacs may be preferred. The information from the audit is most appropriately generalized to the entire agency nursing staff, and it is information about patients already discharged. Also, the descriptions of items, when used in the context of evaluation of a total nursing service, are on a level of generalization that permits the less-than-personalized thinking that attributes measurements to "them." With the Qualpacs, on the other hand, because of the way the data are gathered and the manner of selection of patients whose care is measured, the particular nursing unit from which particular measurements were obtained can be readily identified. Furthermore, the items and, more particularly, the cues are delineated in concrete terms which are readily understood by all categories of personnel. When findings are reported to the staff, specific kinds of care activities can readily be identified by the staff as being attributable to themselves, and they can move directly to planning for changes.

This is not to say that similar kinds of reporting cannot be achieved with either tool. Rather, ready grasping of meaning of the information and recognition of its applicability to themselves is attained by auxiliary staff with information gleaned with the Qualpacs. This does not mean that measurements from Qualpacs will be used to point fingers at individuals; rather, it means that specifics of care provided patients can be readily identified by a unit staff as a whole. The information can serve as specifics for understanding and a basis for immediate planning for improvements in practice.

When decision is made to introduce the administrative component of quality control, there is usually an urgency for getting on with it. There is reluctance to wait for an evolutionary, educational involvement process, which is characteristic in the institutionalization of the Nursing Audit. There is an urgency for finding out about shortcomings and for introducing changes calculated to improve practice. In a fairly short period of time, either tool would furnish information on which to begin planning for improvement. But for a long-range program, there is interest in knowing whether and what differences the changes promote. Since approximately four months is required for an internal audit committee to develop sufficient competence in the use of the audit to ensure reliable measurements, users have frequently elected to use the Qualpacs as the tool for initiation of the program. With it, baseline data can be secured within a relatively short period of time. For example, two nurses could learn to use the scale and have baseline measurements for two to three nursing units in one week of full-time work. Following that, each nurse can secure baseline measurements for at least two units per week. The securing of baseline data with Qualpacs does not commit the agency to sole use of that measuring device for all future measurements; it does serve as a means for having baseline data from which to determine effects of early changes in program.

There can be no delineation of sets of circumstances under which one tool or the other would be chosen. Rather, the foregoing is presented to alert planners to various factors that might appropriately be considered when making tool selection for promotion of the quality control program of a nursing service or for other programs where evaluations of quality of nursing performance or care of patients are needed. In addition to the factors herein identified, the publication of each tool describes experiences that users in varied agencies have had with the tool. These experiences can suggest other elements that may be analogues of those of planners developing quality control, educational, or research programs, and thereby serve as bases for decisions about tool selection for their own situation.

## References

1. Wandelt MA, Slater Stewart D: The Slater Nursing Competencies Rating Scale. New York, Appleton, 1975, p 101
2. Wandelt MA, Ager JW: The Quality Patient Care Scale. New York, Appleton, 1974, p 84

# Chapter 15
# EVALUATION OF PATIENT HEALTH/ WELLNESS OUTCOMES

Marie J. Zimmer, R.N., M.S.N., F.A.A.N.
Norma M. Lang, R.N., Ph.D.

In the history of evaluation of health care for the purpose of assuring society of proper utilization and quality of health care and services, few evaluators measured patient health/wellness outcomes. As a result, current public and voluntary requirements for professional standards or quality assurance review of outcomes necessitate creativity and innovation.

An *outcome* is the health/wellness status of the patient which results from diagnostic, treatment, prognostic, and care activities. Common synonyms for outcome are end result and benefit. In evaluation of health/wellness outcomes, patient functioning on significant variables for the several areas that represent total health, eg, biologic, emotional, social, learning, vocational and avocational behavior,[1] is measured to determine health status. For example, B. Starfield, a physician, proposes a health status evaluation model with seven categories of outcome that have both magnitude and direction and that can be arrayed in parallel.[2] Starfield believes that a profile of patient performance based on the following outcome would describe the health status of individuals, groups of patients, or a population:

Longevity
Activity

Comfort
Satisfaction
Disease
Achievement
Resilience[2]

Sources for information on the subareas of health in which positive change is most frequently caused by nursing activities are Henderson, Kragel et al., Orem, King, and Abdellah et al.[3-7] These and other nursing sources might be studied in conjunction with subareas identified by other physicians such as Sanazaro and Williamson.[8] Although, as Siegel points out, it is difficult to define health,[9] it is important that health care professionals define and use an array of significant elements, such as those identified by Starfield, to guide or classify and report the results of patient health/wellness outcome evaluation.

In professional standards or quality assurance review, in which members of the health care professions take the responsibility individually and collectively to define criteria, standards, and norms, compare the results of practice with these, and take action on the results, serious consideration *must* be given to implementation of an evaluation system that includes monitoring of patient health/wellness outcomes or benefits. An adequate system for care evaluation should provide answers to the questions: "What difference did nursing, medical, pharmacy, social work, or allied health care make in the health status of the patient populations of the institution/agency and community/region? Was the difference the best that the current science and art of each of the professions has to offer? If not, why not? What improvements must be implemented in order to assure society of the best available patient health status end results?"

Maria C. Phaneuf points out in Chapter 1 that evaluation of process and resources *assumes* a relationship between process or resources and outcomes of care. Usually, the relationship to general or specific patient health status outcomes is not known. So, a health care review system that provides only information on use or availability of process and resources provides no concrete information to show that care activities and resources made a difference in the health status of the recipients of care. Furthermore, the data from health care review provides no information that contributes to validation of the assumptions that were made about either the connection between process and patient health/wellness status or the connection of resources to process, followed by the connection of this process to patient health/wellness outcomes. Starfield believes that after mapping of patients' performance for the seven outcome categories that she proposed, the outcome profiles could be used to evaluate the efforts of processes and structure.[2] Advantages can be gained by evaluating outcomes, processes, and structure simultaneously, for then there is knowledge of both the result and the reason for the result. Nevertheless, in health care review, measurement of patient health/wellness outcomes is an essential first step.

The question can be asked: "If evaluation of patient health/wellness outcomes is so important, why is there so little reported work of measurement and evaluation of patient health/wellness benefits?" Chapter 1 gives an array of problems or obstacles that includes the difficulties encountered in definition of end results, the confusing situation caused by the influence of variables other than health care on outcomes, the restriction imposed by the fact that some outcomes may not be known for years, the complexity caused by mobility of people, and the limitations due to an orientation to episodic or disease care and to hospital care. Also, broad definitions of health are generally not operational. In addition, the medical frame of reference constrains definition of the nursing elements. Furthermore, an orientation to the self-image of the discipline rather than to the needs of patients influences the volume of efforts to identify patient benefits or end results versus professional and profession benefits or end results.

Do these and other problems need to cause registered nurses to reject measurement and evaluation of patient health/wellness outcomes? Since the problems can be identified before and during the process of evaluation and since the problem-solving process is a valued part of the armamentarium of nursing skills, it seems that nurses could accept the special challenges inherent in a commitment to measurement and evaluation of patient health/wellness outcomes. The mid-1970s may be an especially opportune time to do so since societal forces such as Professional Standards Review (PSR) legislation and updated standards of voluntary accreditation bodies, such as the Joint Commission on Accreditation of Hospitals (JCAH), have established new requirements. These requirements could help to widen the opening in the door to progress.

# EXPECTATIONS OF ORGANIZATIONS FOR HEALTH CARE REVIEW

Organization of a staff in a health care institution or agency or organization of the members of one or more professional disciplines in a community, region, or state for health care review may be accomplished under a range of program proponents, eg, self-regulation of staff for an institution or agency, Federal Utilization Review Regulations (UR),[10] Federal Professional Standards Review Organizations (PSROs),[10,11] Federal contracts for development work such as Experimental Medical Care Review Organizations (EMCRO),[12] American Hospital Association Quality Assurance Program (QAP),[13] The Joint Commission on Accreditation of Hospitals Performance Evaluation Procedures (PEP),[14,15] and others. In many of these programs, there are commonalities in the purpose and types of review. Usually, the purpose of a health care review organization is to assure the proper quality and utilization of health care services. This is accomplished through three integrated review components: 1) Admission and continued stay certification with a link to discharge planning, 2) health care evaluation studies, and 3) profile analysis.

The purpose of review of *necessity for admission and continued stay*, which is frequently referred to as concurrent review or utilization review (UR), is to determine whether or not admission and continued stay in a particular segment of the health care system is justified by the patient's health status and diagnostic, treatment, prognostic, and care needs. The objective is to ascertain that patients receive care in the least expensive segment of the health care system without jeopardy to the quality of patient benefits. The usual method for implementation is for utilization review coordinators to compare each included patient's diagnosis or problem and supporting data with admission standards. If necessity for admission is established, the coordinator posts the patient's chart with a norm for length of stay for patients with that particular diagnosis or problem. If discharge is not accomplished on or before the norm date, the utilization review coordinator collects record and interview data to determine whether or not data are consistent with one of the exceptions outlined in the standards. Questioned cases of necessity for admission and continued stay are referred to a physician advisor for a clinical decision.

A strong relationship between length of stay and discharge planning is assumed. The standards for monitoring of continued stay may include benchmarks for monitoring staff's attention to and progress in development, with the patient and significant others, of a care plan for posthospital or post-skilled nursing home care. The benchmarks may be tied to time, eg, admission day, third hospital day, or at discharge.

*Health Care Evaluation (HCE) studies,* which are frequently referred to as retrospective reviews or audits, are for the purpose of determining whether or not care meets the proper standard of quality as defined by professionals. The objective is to ascertain that persons receive care commensurate with the best available knowledge. The usual method for implementation is for peer groups from the specialty area to define the process and/or outcome standards for diagnosis, treatment, prognosis, and care for a very specific patient population and to specify the sample of completed records for patients with that diagnosis, problem, or treatment that is to be reviewed. Specialists screen medical records by comparing data in the records with the standards, and present the findings to a review group with members not personally involved with care for that particular population. This review group evaluates the records of care for patients in which there is variation from the standard, evaluates these and other data, makes recommendations, and prepares a report of the study for the appropriate body, eg, an audit committee which in turn reports, through designated channels, to the appropriate persons and bodies, such as the director of services, administration, and hospital board.

Health care professionals are expected to identify priority areas for health care evaluation studies. Goran and colleagues, in a discussion of PSRO HCE, stated, "Their (HCES) subject matter varies greatly and can include review of the patient care process, patient outcomes, the use of a given procedure, or the operating characteristics of an institution."[16] Probable problem areas should rank high on the priority list.

*Profile analysis* is used to monitor the effectiveness of reviews of necessity for admission and continued stay and health care evaluation studies. From large pools of data, conclusions are to be drawn about patterns of care in the institution or agency and community or region, and priorities for future reviews are to be recommended. Necessarily, profile analysis must follow implementation of the other two types of review because it is dependent on these for pooled data.

An important resource for a regionalized health review network is a data system that can pool specific groups of data that are developed and reported from a number of settings in the region. For example, the National Professional Standards Review Council (NPSRC) is studying the need for a minimum basic data set for use in PSROs. Health System Agencies (HSA) are also concerned about data sets and systems. Nurses need to know and comply with the data sets and system that are adopted for their particular agency or institution.

The three types of review are intended to function as an integrated system. Findings from one type of review can impact on another type and change the priority rank for studies in that area. For example, if the hospital stay for an extensive number of patients in a specific population is extended beyond the norm because of febrile states, the UR body might recommend a HCE study to etablish the causative factors. Also, specific studies may be comprehensive. For example, a HCE study may determine whether or not admission and discharge UR standards were met in addition to the primary focus of the study on proper care and outcomes for the period of care. UR is a review of individual cases. HCES might include review of patterns of utilization for a sample of a population.

*PSRO Program Manual* guidelines encourage peer groups to develop complete sets of standards from which subsets can be drawn for specific purpose reviews.[17] A complete set would then contain standards for admission, health status outcomes at specific points in time, eg, at discharge, and perhaps elements in the process of care that are critical to proper health status outcomes and appropriate use of resources.

One advantage of scaled measurement instruments is that for each variable, nurses can determine which descriptor best depicts the necessity for admission to the particular segment of the health care delivery system. Then nurses can determine which descriptor for each variable best represents desired health/wellness at discharge to the next segment of the health care delivery system. These choices are the nursing standards for necessity for admission and health/wellness outcomes at discharge. For review of necessity for continued stay, the negative variations from the discharge standards are the justifications of necessity for continued stay. In this way, nurses can develop complete sets of standards from which subsets can be drawn as needed.

Physicians, administrators, and fiscal intermediaries may interpret failure of nurses to participate in one or more types of review to mean that nursing makes no important contributions. For example, if nurses do not provide standards for necessity for admission to a particular segment of the health care delivery system, eg, a hospital, for inclusion with the set developed by physicians, the omission may be interpreted to mean that nurses have no standards to draw upon for the decision of whether or not the patient should be admitted. Furthermore, if registered nurses do not provide the standards, someone else may. For example, during a continued stay review, the utilization review coordinator may collect data from records or interviews of nurses. In the absence of standards from nurses for comparison with the nurses' data, physician advisors may use a self-defined standard and make the decision about necessity.

Health care review is oriented to populations and groups. It is monitoring of care for patient populations, not individual patients. Currently, admission certification, which is closely tied to authorization for payment by the fiscal intermediary, appears to be an exception. However, in the future populations for which necessity for admission is more clear cut, eg, delivery of a baby, may be excepted. Health care review is also monitoring of the practice of the group of practitioners such as, the registered nurses who care for a cardiovascular surgery patient population, not individual practitioners.

Although the task of planning, developing, and implementing nursing health care review is arduous, and although it may be tempting to concentrate on one type of review, eg, retrospective studies of patient health/wellness outcomes at discharge, nurses should be contributing to each of the three types of review.

# FUNCTIONS OF THE NURSE IN HEALTH CARE REVIEW

For health care review, registered nurses are expected to first of all establish criteria, standards, and norms. Frequently, communication is hampered by lack of uniform definition of terms, and nurses should know the definitions used by colleagues and organizations under whose aegis the program operates. For PSRO definitions see the PSRO Program Manual.[17] For definitions used by other organizations, check their manuals.

*Criteria* refer to the kinds of variables or elements that are to be assessed. When the objective for evaluation is to monitor patient health/wellness outcomes, only the criterion variables that are the most significant or critical elements of the health/wellness status for a specific patient population are selected. After each significant element is identified, the range of different patient health attributes that fully describe patients' health/wellness status on the variable are identified. From the full range of attributes, those that are assumed or known to be the most powerful indicators of patient functioning on the variable are selected for use in monitoring quality. Those that are selected are graduated to show more than two levels of magnitude of that attribute. Scales for use in measurement are a result.

*Standard* refers to the level of magnitude that must be achieved on each scale in order to make a qualitative statement about the goodness of the patient health/wellness outcomes. This may be expressed as a constant, for example, patients should reach point 3 on a specific scale prior to discharge to home care, or as a range, for example, at discharge 80 percent of the patients should reach point 5 on the scale and because of intervening variables, 20 percent may reach points 3 or

4. Desirably, a range such as this would be derived from the results of studies of a specific patient population so that the statistics were supported by empirical data rather than estimates.

Usually, the peer group has a very specific aim when the members express a range for acceptable variation. A range may take into account intervening variables that impact on patients' progress toward health/wellness, eg, secondary diagnosis, or ability to function in another segment of the health care delivery system, eg, distance or support from family unit. In the JCAH method, the standard is always set at 100 percent or 0 percent. The aim is to alert the medical records personnel of what must be documented in the patients' record.[18] All variations are examined by the peer group.

Since a patient's health status as measured with the scale varies over time, standards are usually tied to time, eg, at discharge or two months posthospitalization. Professional intramural and extramural peer groups use their experience and the recommendations of experts and make judgments about the appropriate standards.

A *norm* is a statistical measure that is derived empirically from a large pool of data. If nurses from 29 different institutions used the same variables and pooled their HCES findings for 29 subpopulations of the total regional population of adult, newly-diagnosed, insulin-dependent patients with diabetes mellitus not secondary to another diagnosis or treatment regimen, the profile of norms for a set of variables might be calculated, if there was not too much variability in the study findings.

Specialty disciplinary peer groups in institutions and agencies are expected to establish their standards and to contribute to development of norms. They are also expected to form a coalition with members of other disciplines to form interdisciplinary sets of criteria, standards, and norms. In regional reviews, the source for standards might be a committee of a health review organization, a specialty group in an organization for the specific profession, a contract with a group in a university, and so on.

For health care review, registered nurses are also expected to establish mechanisms to review care and to conduct reviews.[19,20] One good source of information is the system for review described by Maria C. Phaneuf for audit of process standards. Systems recommended by government, accrediting agencies, and professional and health delivery associations are other good sources. Users should evaluate these review systems before adopting one for use. The JCAH, for example, requires a health review system to have six characteristics:

1. *Valid* criteria that permit objective review of the *quality* of care provided to *all* patients are established.
2. *Measurement* of actual practice against the criteria produces *reliable* data.
3. *Results* of measurement are *analyzed* by peers.
4. *Action* is taken to correct the *problems* identified.
5. Action is *followed up.*
6. The results of patient care, that is, general findings and specific recommendations, are *reported.* [21]

Nurses are expected to develop mechanisms for use of findings from HCEs and URs. Although evaluation of variations from standards and norms may yield recommendations for a wide range of improvement actions to be implemented by a variety of persons in the setting, it is expected that a considerable number of recommendations will concern continuing education. Jesse and collaborators describe continuing education expectations of providers and three different levels in the PSRO organization. [22] In the future, staff development educators will find that the need for specific continuing education programs will be identified in the recommendations from health care reviews, and the long-term results of continuing education programs will be determined through HCE restudies.

The establishment of valid criteria and standards that permit objective review of the quality of care provided to patients is a basic step in most review systems. The selection of the type of criteria depends on the purpose for the review and the kind of information to be gathered. What is to be evaluated? The institution? The nurses? The patients? All three are important in the delivery of quality nursing services. Is the purpose of the review to satisfy review requirements by some outside governmental or accrediting agency? Or is the purpose to obtain information that is useful in making decisions about the improvement of nursing care? Or, are both purposes appropriate?

When developing criteria, consideration is given to the clarification of values held regarding health and medical care. It is impossible to discuss quality without examining values of the professional, the client, and the health organization. Most conflicts about quality care arise between those holding different values. Although values are the real determinants of quality, it is difficult to make these values explicit. Written criteria are clear or explicit statements of values and beliefs held regarding quality patient care.

When establishing a review system, it is helpful to decide on a model or framework to guide activities. A framework might include the following components or steps:

1. Clarification of values

2. Establishment of outcome, process and structure standards, and criteria for nursing care
3. Assessment of the degree of discrepancy between the standards and criteria and the current level of nursing practice
4. Selection and implementation of an alternative for changing nursing practice
5. Improvement of nursing practice[23]

This type of framework clearly points out the purpose of the review to be the improvement of nursing practice. The framework indicates that criteria are to be developed based upon the current values. Finally, the framework provides for the data collected about current nursing practice to serve as a basis for decision making regarding changes in nursing practice. A similar type of model or framework, along with guidelines for its implementation, can be found in a recent report released by the American Nurses' Association, Committee on Implementation of Standards.[24]

# HOW OUTCOME CRITERIA ARE DEVELOPED

If the decision is made to measure quality nursing services with a focus on patient health/wellness outcomes, then outcome criteria must be developed. Patient health/wellness outcome criteria are the elements of the health status which are to be measured. Positive indices can be used in assessing the alteration in the consumer's health status. Examples are an increase in patients' health knowledge, ability to function in work and personal roles, and ability to maintain positive health behavior. Assessment of the outcomes of nursing care can also be measured using negative indices. Examples are failure to maintain or improve patients' health status, disability, discomfort, and complications.[25]

Outcome criteria are usually written for a specific group of patients. These can be of a general nature for a large target patient population. An example is the set suggested by the Association of Operating Room Nurses for all patients having surgery:

The individual is free from infection.

The individual's skin integrity is maintained.

The individual is free of adverse effects from lack of or improper use of safety measures; improper position; extraneous objects; chemical, physical, and electrical hazards.

The individual's fluid and electrolyte balance is maintained.

The individual demonstrated knowledge of his physiologic and psychologic responses to surgical intervention. [26]

Outcome criteria can also be written for specific patient populations. The determination of patient populations presents a challenge to nurses. The most frequent grouping currently being used in nursing review is that of medical diagnosis or problem. For example, a set of outcome criteria is written for patients with congestive heart failure. Most institutions use medical diagnosis as the method of classification of patients for admission, discharge, staffing, and record-retrieval. Therefore, it is reasonable for most staffs to use medical diagnosis as the classification for review. Other classifications or groupings, however, may be more meaningful to nurses. These are such classifications as nursing diagnosis, nursing problems, and developmental status. For example, nurses may choose to develop criteria for patients who are immobilized, patients who are hyperactive, or the well three-month-old infant. Patient classifications that are relevant, useable, and retrievable should be used.

The selections of patient populations are made after an examination of the most frequently occurring diagnoses or problems in a specific institution or practice. Little useful information can be gained from the selection of a patient diagnosis or problem which rarely occurs.

The patient population may require further limitation in order to make criteria most consistent and meaningful. Additional patient characteristics which may be used are the patient's sex, age, severity of problem, language ability, and geographic location. Government and organizations have specific requirements regarding number and kind of patients to be reviewed. These requirements are also given consideration when selecting patient populations. For example, PSRO requires reviews of all patients receiving Medicaid, Medicare, and Maternal-Child Health benefits.

A set of outcome criteria is developed for each selected patient population. After significant elements are identified, the range of different health attributes that fully describe the patient's health/wellness status on the variable are identified. These critiera are scaled or graduated to show more than two levels of magnitude of that attribute. The following are examples of scaled criteria for a population of adult patients who are immobilized and hospitalized. [27] For the variables of circulation and bowel elimination, three scales are the following:

| Scale #1 | Scale #2 | Scale #3 |
|---|---|---|
| 3 plus edema of lower extremity at rest | Severe cramping with movement of lower extremity | Impaction requiring digital removal |
| 2 plus edema of lower extremity at rest | Mild pain with movement of lower extremity | Irregular bowel evacuation requiring mechanical or chemical stimulation |
| 1 plus edema of lower extremity at rest | Pain on calf compression | Regular bowel evacuation requiring mechanical or chemical stimulation |
| Absence of edema of lower extremity at rest | Absence of pain in lower extremity | Regular bowel evacuation with dietary control |

A set of outcome criteria can also be written with a specific time for achievement. This time is usually referred to as the critical time. If scaled criteria are available, a single point on the scale can be selected for the standard at a specific time. Examples of criteria with a critical time are listed in Table 1.

When nurses begin to develop sets of outcome critieria, it is helpful to examine sample sets of criteria. Examples of outcome criteria are

### Table 1

### Patient Population: Patients having an Abdominal Hysterectomy, Age 20-40

| Criterion | Critical time |
|---|---|
| Patient demonstrates coughing and deep breathing exercise. | Preoperative |
| Patient stayed in bed unless assisted. | 24 hours postoperative |
| Respiratory rate between 16 and 26. | 24 hours postoperative |
| Patient demonstrates self-examination of the breast. | Time of discharge |
| Incision is clean and dry. | Time of discharge |
| Patient names medications which she is taking home. | Time of discharge |

Outcome criteria can be written for a specific patient population for a specific developmental stage. The following are examples[23]:

**Patient Population:  Healthy three-month-old infant who has been seen by a Pediatric Nurse Practitioner since birth**

Criteria

Infant maintains birth percentile in weight.
Infant vocalizes other than crying.
Infant sleeps 7 to 10 hr through the night.
Infant has consistent caretakers.
Infant's mother has pursued, or is planning to pursue, activities
    outside of the home not related to her infant.
Infant has received primary immunizations.

beginning to appear in nursing literature.[15,28-35] A major contract to develop criteria for measuring the quality and effectiveness of nursing care was awarded to the American Nurses' Association (ANA).[36] As a result of the contract, the ANA developed prototype sets of outcome criteria for specific patient populations within the medical-surgical, maternal-child, psychiatric-mental health, community health, and gerontologic nursing practice areas. Nurses should examine the results of this project for assistance in the development and use of outcome criteria and standards.

# WHO DEVELOPS OUTCOME CRITERIA

The question arises as to who should develop outcome criteria. Nurses who are practicing or actually delivering the nursing care are in the best position to determine which criteria are to be used. Peer groups of nurses should establish the sets of criteria. Clinical specialists have a responsibility to share their expertise in terms of outcome criteria for their specialty populations. Consideration must be given to documenting the selected criteria utilizing the results of nursing research as found in nursing literature. Validity of criteria will be strengthened when peer groups of nurses seek agreement on sets of outcome criteria. Administrative and educator nurses can facilitate and assist the practitioners as they meet the task of developing criteria.

# HOW OUTCOME CRITERIA ARE USED

The overall purpose of developing health/wellness outcome criteria and standards is to use them to measure and improve the nursing care delivered to clients/patients. When outcome criteria are used, the quality of nursing care is measured by the results of that care. When the criteria are placed in a measurement tool, the strengths and weaknesses of a nursing practice can be determined. In other words, the degree of achievement of the criteria is determined. This information is then used as a basis for making a change in the practice of nursing.

More specifically, a set of outcome criteria can be used in a nursing audit. The Joint Commission on the Accreditation of Hospitals recommends that a set of outcome criteria, with the critical time at the patient's discharge, be used to evaluate the care of a group of patients. The Commission further recommends that a retrospective audit of records be the method utilized to collect the information. If patient's progress on criterion variables is not documented in the record, then the process of nursing care should be examined and methods for improvement of the care carried out. Reaudit should then demonstrate an improvement in care.

The PSRO groups recommend that screening outcome criteria can be used to examine the care of large numbers of patients. Screening criteria are a selected few critical criteria which can be applied to review of care for a large number of patients. Patients' records "falling through the screen" then need to be examined using a larger number of in-depth outcome or process criteria. The patient record is the usual repository of information that is used in PSRO reviews. Occasionally, direct contact is made with the patient or the nurse for information, particularly for concurrent admission and continued stay review.

One outcome criterion can serve as an illustration of how nursing care can be improved. For a patient population of women, age 20 to 40 years who have had an abdominal hysterectomy, the following outcome criterion was established: The patient demonstrates self-examination of the breast. The critical time is at discharge from the hospital.

This criterion was seated in a retrospective record audit, and 50 patient records were audited. Not one record was found to have documented the achievement or nonachievement of this criterion. The nurses involved in the practice reaffirmed that this criterion was descriptive of quality patient care. Several discussions ensued including one in which it was determined that the hospital philosophy did not include wellness-type care because of the related expense. Some administrative persons felt that if the abdominal incision was clean and dry, the patient afebrile, and the patient ambulatory, that these were sufficient criteria. Patient instruction in health care practices was a bonus, not an essential. The values of the nurses and the values of the administration were in conflict. Much discussion was required before the administrators began to acknowledge a responsibility for selected aspects of health teaching. The nurses then instituted a plan to teach all patients within the target population how to do a self-examination of the breast. Before discharge, patients were asked to demonstrate this technique, and the results were recorded in the discharge summary. The next audit using this criterion yielded a 75 percent achievement. This simple illustration serves as an example of how outcome criteria can be utilized to improve nursing practice.

Outcome criteria can also be utilized in tools which involve direct observation of patients. Some authorities feel that direct observation and interview of the patient has more reliability than a review of the records. Others believe that the method of direct observation is too expensive for most institutions to utilize at all times.

Outcome criteria can be utilized in patient self-rating questionnaires. Frequently, questionnaires to patients asking them to evaluate the care received elicit only a satisfaction-type response. Outcome criteria placed in a self-rating questionnaire has the potential of determining the patient's perspective of his achievement on the criteria.

Educators in undergraduate, graduate, and continuing education programs are viewing outcome criteria as a means of planning and evaluating curriculum and program offerings. A set of outcome criteria for a specific patient population can serve as an organizing framework for the teaching of care of that population. By continually predicting where the patient should be on each criterion variable, students are assisted in evaluating the individual care of patients as well as groups of patients. Staff development leaders are looking to the criteria development and measurement as a means of identifying continuing education and in-service needs of nurses. In time, these criteria may serve to evaluate the educational program as well.

The challenge of outcome criteria has also been accepted by nurse researchers who are attempting to identify the most valid and reliable predictors or indicators of quality nursing care.

# CHALLENGE FOR THE FUTURE

The answer to the question, "What is Quality Nursing?" is not easy or complete. The answer will constantly be changing as scientific knowledge, values, and resources change. A continual look at the structure, process, and outcome parameters of patient care is required. Additional studies on each parameter of patient care plus the relationships of all three, ie, cause and effect studies, will help determine the best nursing care practices.

A sharing of studies and reviews by nurses in the literature will help to accelerate better answers to the question of quality. Workshops and other educational programs can assist more nurses in the methodologies of reviews.

Outcome criteria need to be tested further for validity and reliability. Currently, most outcome criteria that are used have only content or face validity, which means there is a peer consensus regarding the importance and relevance of the criteria. Additional studies will help nurses to learn more about the best predictors of the relationship of nursing practice to resolution of patient health/wellness problems.

Patient health/wellness outcome criteria are indicators of the status of the patient. They show the end result of diagnostic, treatment, prognostic, and care activities. The establishment and utilization of criteria is one of the most important challenges facing the nursing profession today. It would be well for every professional nurse to become involved in the decision making about criteria and standards that will describe quality nursing care to the public.

## References

1.  Platron KC, Brophy JJ: Review of areas/A key to diagnosis. *Postgraduate Medicine* 42:A137-A141, 1967
2.  Starfield B: Measurement of outcome: a proposed scheme. Milbank Memorial Fund Quarterly: Health and Society. Winter 1974, pp 41–45
3.  Henderson V: ICN Basic Principles of Patient Care. Geneva, Switzerland, International Council of Nurses, 1960
4.  Kragel JM, Mousseau VS, Goldsmith C, Arora R: Patient Care Systems. Philadelphia, Lippincott, 1974, pp 11–20
5.  Orem DE: Nursing Concepts of Practice. New York, McGraw-Hill, 1971
6.  King IM: Toward a Theory for Nursing: General Concepts of Human Behavior. New York, Wiley, 1971
7.  Abdellah FG, Beland IL, Martin A, Matheney RV: Patient-centered Approaches to Nursing. New York, MacMillan, 1969
8.  Sanazaro PJ, Williamson JW: Physician performance and its effect on patients: a classification based on reports by internists, surgeons, pediatricians, and obstetricians. Medical Care 8:2, 299–308
9.  Siegel H: To your health—whatever that may mean. Nursing Forum 12:3, 281–89
10.  Public Law 92-603.
11.  Office of Professional Standards Review. PSRO Program Manual. Washington, D.C., U.S. Department of Health, Education and Welfare, March 15, 1974
12.  National Center for Health Services Research and Development. Ex-

perimental Medical Care Review Organization (EMCRO) Program. Washington, D.C., Department of Health, Education and Welfare, March, 1973 DHEW Publication No. (HSM) 73-3017

13. American Hospital Association. Quality Assurance Program for Medical Care in the Hospital. Chicago, American Hospital Association, 1972
14. Joint Commission on Accreditation of Hospitals. Accreditation Manual for Hospitals. Chicago, 1972
15. Smith AP: PEP Workbook for Nurses. Chicago, Joint Commission on Accreditation of Hospitals, 1974
16. Goran MJ, Roberts JS, Kellogg M, Fielding J, Jesse W: The PSRO hospital review system. Medical Care 13(4):17, April 1975
17. Office of Professional Standards Review. pp 18–19
18. Greeley HP, Stearns G: Primer on Retrospective Outcome Audit. Quality Review Bulletin 1(1):6–9, September 1974
19. Zimmer MJ: A Model for Evaluating Nursing Care. Hospitals 48(5)91–95, 131, March 1, 1974
20. Zimmer MJ: Quality Assurance for Nursing Care. Proceedings of an Institute Jointly Sponsored by the American Nurses' Association and the American Hospital Association, October 29–31, 1973. Kansas City, American Nurses' Association, 1974
21. Joint Commission on Accreditation of Hospitals. Perspective on Accreditation: Special Supplement. January–February 1975
22. Jesse WF, Munier WB, Fielding JE, Goran MJ: PSRO: an educational force for improving quality of care. New Engl J of Med 292(13): 668–71
23. Lang NL: A Model for Quality Assurance in Nursing. Unpublished doctoral dissertation, Marquette University, 1974
24. American Nurses' Association, Congress for Nursing Practice. Report of the ad hoc Advisory Committee for Implementation of Standards of Nursing Practice, Kansas City, Mo., 1975
25. Wisconsin Regional Medical Program Nursing Committee. Quality assurance in nursing care: a position paper. Stat. Bulletin of the Wisconsin Nurses' Association 42(3)10–11 March 1973. Reprinted in Nursing Digest 2(8):79–81, October 1974
26. Association of Operating Room Nurses. Nursing Audit: Challenge to the Operating Room Nurse. Denver, Association of Operating Room Nurses, 1974
27. Zimmer M, Lang NL, Miller D: Development of Sets of Patient Health Outcome Criteria by Panels of Nurse Experts. Madison, Wisconsin Regional Medical Program, 1974
28. Quality Review Bulletin. Chicago, Joint Commission on Accreditation of Hospitals, Quality Review Center, 1975–76
29. Zimmer JJ et al: Guidelines for development of outcome criteria. Nursing Clinics of North America, June 1974
30. Bloch D: Evaluation of nursing care in terms of process and outcomes. Nursing Research 24(4):256–63, July–August 1975
31. Hegyvary S, Chamings P: The hospital setting and patient care outcomes. Journal of Nursing Service Administration, May 1975
32. Hilger EE: Developing nursing outcome criteria. Nursing Clinics of North America, June 1974
33. Anderson MI: Development of outcome criteria for the patient with congestive heart failure. Nursing Clinics of North America, June 1974

34.  Taylor JW: Measuring the outcomes of nursing care. Nursing Clinics of North America, June 1974
35.  Division of Nursing. A Methodology for Monitoring Quality of Nursing Care. Washington, D.C., DHEW Publication No. (HRA) 74-75, U.S. Department of Health, Education and Welfare, January 1974
36.  American Nurses' Association. PSRO contract awarded to develop care criteria. American Nurse 6(1), September 1974

# Chapter **16**
## REFLECTIONS

## AN END TO STRUCTURE VERSUS PROCESS VERSUS OUTCOME DEBATES?

Optimal self-regulation in nursing practice and collaboration with other disciplines so that patients, families, and the public can ultimately be assured of quality care wherever service is provided will not be achieved until debates about the importance of structure versus process versus outcome have been ended and replaced by acceptance of each of the components as essential to the larger whole presently projected as "quality assurance."

With regard to effectiveness, structure requires more attention than it is presently receiving. Morse et al have suggested that a set of criteria for an "effective" hospital should be developed—effectiveness meaning the capacity to deliver high-quality patient care.[1] Search of the literature has not yielded any such criterion sets for other health care facilities, either. Criteria for evaluation are of major importance here, because features of organizational structures "derive their significance from a system of values that needs to be made explicit so that it can be subjected to scrutiny."[2]

Similarly, the structural aspects of quality assurance systems require sets of criteria pertinent to effectiveness, of which cost-effectiveness is an element. As mentioned previously, quality assurance viewed on a general systems theory base requires that "structure," "process," and "outcome" be considered components in the system and that, for each component, there are some methods in use that deal primarily with that component and are addressed to total populations served, and other methods that are addressed to selected populations at special clinical risks or of special concern for other reasons.

Two criteria proposed for evaluation of organizations are presented here to illustrate the way in which evaluation criteria directed to effectiveness are equally applicable to quality assurance systems.

The criterion of control over key organizational (system) functions and processes is subject to the following:

1. Control only as justified by legitimate organizational objectives, not simply accumulating power
2. Minimum controls necessary to achieve organizational objectives
3. Maximum internalization of controls through education, socialization, and linkage with basic professional and social values
4. Maximum reliance on positive incentives and minimum reliance on negative sanctions[2]

The second criterion deals with assessment as necessary to rational planning, operation, and control of the organization (system). Major attributes of the assessment process are the following:

1. It is continuing.
2. It is systematized by virtue of having several components that are interrelated and mutually reinforcing rather than being an assemblage of random, ad hoc activities.
3. It includes monitoring of the outcomes as well as the process of care.
4. It is linked to action, so that deviations from expected performance result in investigation and appropriate action, which is preventive and rehabilitative, rather than mainly punitive.
5. It preferably has external, in addition to internal, components.
6. It is formalized, but it is supported by many informal features of the organization (system) and by shared values and objectives.[2]

## One Attack on the Malpractice Problem: Personalizing Care

The importance of personalizing care has hitherto been presented as part of the quality of care to which patients, and family members or other persons important to the patient and to whom the patient is important, are entitled. Personalizing care is also structurally important for the protection of health care facilities, cost containment here included. The cost of malpractice insurance coverage has risen to the point that it is beginning to be directly reflected in per diem cost of hospital care, as well as in physicians' fees.[3] This is in addition to the increase in costs related to laboratory and other procedures used in the practice of defensive medicine (practice designed to assure, as much as possible, successful legal defense in case of suit). The Report of the Secretary's Commission on Medical Malpractice recommends

... (that) continuing programs of research and analysis aimed at increasing knowledge and understanding of patients' psychological and psychosocial needs and the findings of such research be translated into specific action programs, aimed at improving the physical design and methods of management of health care facilities and at improving the training of health-care personnel in the human relations aspects of patient care.[4]

The Commission "fully recognized the importance of the professional nurse in patient care and recommended that physicians, hospitals, nursing homes, and other institutions increase the number of professional nurses giving direct care to patients in the interests of better patient care and of minimizing malpractice suits."[4] The Commission expressed the belief that all hospital employees, especially nurses, should have an understanding of psychology and the art of human relations in order to enhance patient satisfaction and prevent complaints.[4] Another recommendation was that clinical courses which include human anatomy, psychology, and human relations be required in the nursing curriculum.[4] Nursing curricula have for some years included these components; the question is how well the related knowledge is applied, and whether the structures of institutions and agencies impede or facilitiate application of nursing knowledge and understandings in behalf of patients.

In its own way, the Commission appeared aware of the nature of nursing practice. It has added cogency and urgency to the need for retrospective nursing process auditing that includes specific attention to the psychosocial aspects of care and is used to appraise the quality of care received by total populations from unabstracted patient care records. In abstracting, psychosocial components are usually omitted. In any case, the total recorded nursing interventions are needed if a fair view of the nursing process applied is to be obtained on audit.

At best, the retrospective audit would be used by all the care facilities in a given geographic region to help assure the public that, in all facilities in the area, the quality of nursing care is being monitored against common standards. The regional approach would help to focus and consolidate well-aimed continuing education programs for nurses and other workers responsible to nurses; the programs could be designed to meet needs identified through auditing. Most importantly, use of successively developed quality profiles in each health care facility would identify impacts of continuing education on competency in practice.

Regional quality profiles, developed over time, would facilitate identification of staffing needs and problems of quality care related to staffing patterns and monitoring the impacts of change patterns on care received by patients.

With a regional approach, it would also be possible to appraise the quality of care received by the substantial number of specific patients who move to and fro among hospitals, home care, nursing homes, ambulatory services or other care facilities. In this event, not only could the process of care provided to the same patients in different settings be appraised; the outcomes of care for these patients at the end of each institutional/agency cycle of service would then be open to scrutiny.

# NURSING: POTENTIAL CONTRIBUTION TO DEVELOPMENT OF QUALITY APPRAISAL METHODS IN OTHER DISCIPLINES

Physicians have shown interest in the nursing audit from its inception. Some physicians have participated in orientations to the audit and have used its conceptual framework in reexamining medical audit methods. Some social workers and clinical pharmacists have undertaken use of the audit framework, using their own professional content.[5] Nutritionists and physical therapists have expressed interest in using the same approach. One observation arising from all such contacts is that the nursing focus on practice was seen by these social workers, pharmacists, nutritionists, and physical therapists as more congruent with their focus of practice than is the medical approach. If this focus is broadly accepted, it has some high potentials for advancement toward the goal of patient care audits, in which each type of professional participating in care is responsible for appraising the quality of the specific care given and the results synthesized in a true patient care quality appraisal. The possibility that the congruence is real suggests the need for nursing to publicize widely all of its self-regulatory efforts as well as its various quality appraisal methods so that other disciplines may benefit from them. In collegial exchanges at the practice and other levels, nursing has much to offer and much to learn through such exchanges. The public, as well as the professions, ultimately benefits.

# NURSING: POTENTIAL CONTRIBUTION TO CONSUMER PARTICIPATION IN QUALITY ASSURANCE

Consumers, by definition, include us all. By selective definition, the term is applied to people who are not employed in health services.

Despite the problems involved in defining what a health consumer is, and determining who can speak for him, there are two primary concepts on which most people can agree: he has the right to high quality accessible and reasonably priced health services; and he ought to be able to have something to say about the planning and delivery of such services.[6]

Hopefully, we are moving toward the day when evaluation of quality is methodologically built into the planning and delivery of health services.

Division of the health service world into providers and consumers is unfortunate to the extent that such division connotes that providers bestow and consumers use up, and that their goals vary in accordance with the designations. This makes it difficult to move away from the past in which the voice of the patient (he complies, he obeys) was little heard unless he held some power in the situation that derived from his social or economic status. The division makes it difficult to move away from a past in which some communities and parts of communities have been poorly served by the providers of care.[7]

Because nursing is in the vanguard in work toward quality assurance as a part of self-regulation, it is in an uncommonly good position to involve consumers in a contributing way to the development of a climate of earned consumer trust. This means that at local, state, and national levels, consumers should be helped to become knowledgeable about what is being done in their behalf—the ethical bases for action, the goals, the methods used, and overall results. Consumer response should be elicited and suggestions considered and used as feasible. Mechanisms for on-going provider-consumer collaboration would of course be required. Use of consumer advisory committees would be one practical way of honoring consumers' rights. If such committees are established, conceptual frameworks should be developed and specify authorities and responsibilities entailed in committee function.

# NURSING: SOME RESEARCH POTENTIALS RELATED TO QUALITY ASSURANCE

Nursing methods that produce quantitative and descriptive findings of substance will raise innumerable questions that require new knowledge before sound answers can be developed. Identification and delineation of such questions are a part of the performance of process and outcome audits. Many of the questions so identified will fit into the list of items identified by nurse administrators as having highest research priority in terms of potential impact on patient welfare. Educators are also in general agreement with the administrators' identifications.[8]

The need for development of effectiveness criteria for institutions and agencies has been mentioned previously. This area is one in which new knowledge is likely to be required prior to critera development, partly because of the historic pattern of emphasis on efficiency. The pattern is particularly conspicuous in nursing.

The development of quality predictors that would link the process and outcome dimensions of appraisal without destroying the integrity of either would be a breakthrough of stunning proportions not only for nursing, but for health care generally.

Efforts to elicit evaluations of care from patients are now made in most settings. Search of the literature and personal inquiry in approximately 50 hospitals suggests that new knowledge is needed before practical, reliable, and valid instruments that focus on the quality of care as perceived by the patients or the families are developed. Reference has already been made to the serious problem of malpractice suits. What is equally serious, but ignored because there is no direct impact on providers, is the fact that falsely based satisfaction can be expressed by patients. This is apparent in situations in which patients feel that their worth and dignity are respected, and perhaps because of lack of knowledge, they do not recognize that scientific and technical aspects of the care are deplorable by even minimum standards. While the importance of personalizing care in its psychosocial dimension has been necessarily stressed, it is no less recognized that compassionate but clinically unsound care can kill a patient. He may die feeling loved, but he dies.

Research leading to methods of reliable and valid patient and family evaluations of care received should have high priority. Patient care evaluation will not be what the words imply until the patients' view of care is included.

Another area for research germane to self-regulation and practice is the ethos of nursing. Research is urgent here if nursing is to make explicit its present ethical base and precisely examine the morality of its words and actions. Such research might lead to the development of ethicists who are nurses. This does not mean nurse-ethicists, but ethicists whose nursing background would qualify them to be authorities on the application of ethics to nursing education, practice, and research.

Some nurses who are qualified researchers might choose to venture into the area of quality assurance. This area includes assistance in development and evaluation of systems of quality assurance in the application of available nursing methods, development of better methods, and in the continuing development of methods involving other disciplines. Researchers with whom this possibility has been discussed have expressed interest and volunteered recognition of the prior need to have a broad context knowledge of quality assurance history, trends, issues, programs, and methods, to avoid the risk of too narrow a focus for their efforts.

# NURSES: THE GREAT POTENTIAL

More than 20 years of work toward excellence in nursing and health care leaves little doubt that nurses in the United States and Canada are ready, willing, and able to go forward in quality assurance for the benefit of patients, the public, and for the advancement of practice. Reflections from experience may be useful here.

One of the comments repeated over and over again was, "The audit tells that we are better than we thought we were, even if we do have a long way to go." This says something about nurses' self-images that is distressing, because to underestimate ourselves is no less destructive of potentials of individuals and professions than is overestimation. Underestimation may be another manifestation of the influence of the traditional subservient role of women to which women and women as nurses have been socialized. In any event, nurses apparently welcome the opportunity to find out for themselves what indeed is the quality of the service they provide.

If formative evaluation is to yield results in nursing self-esteem, the involvement of staff nurses in the use of nursing methods of quality appraisal is essential. Their involvement is essential for other obvious reasons, including the fact that they provide or are immediately responsible for patient care, and that changes in the direction of quality improvement cannot occur without their participation and leadership.

Perhaps because of our apprenticeship heritage, our previous task and activity orientation, and traditional emphasis on not taking risks, particularly the risk of any kind of error, we as nurses sometimes seem overeager for specific blueprints that will guide nursing practice. The present proliferation of nursing protocols and of protocols that are really algorithms (protocols in which each step is literally contingent on the preceding step), enchantment with computers and automated systems, and love-hate reactions to criteria development may reflect this need for blueprints. This is not to say that protocols, criteria, and whatever technology is available or can be developed should not be used, because they should be used to the maximum. The maximum use, however, is to assist nurses to carry on the practice of nursing as an intellectual discipline, and to do so effectively and efficiently. Care should be patient-oriented, and not computer-oriented or protocol-oriented. The other nagging notion that lurks in the mind is the possibility that, when we put undue effort in working with things, we avoid or postpone examination of nurse-patient interactions, even though we know that conscious use of self lies in the core of professional practice.

These observations connote only the risk that some nursing potentials may be lost if we make injudicious use of assistive devices of whatever nature and in so doing lose sight of the patient, or groups of patients, as human beings and lose sight of ourselves as professionals who are human beings.

The risk of lost potentials is relatively small; the majority of nurses care about the people they take care of, and about nursing. The caring has been amply demonstrated by positive responses to the rigors of the nursing audit, including eagerness for self-renewal in themselves and nursing.

## UNITY IN NURSING: THE DESIDERATUM?

Self-regulation in nursing practice, with a special focus on appraisal of the quality of nursing care, can be the moral ground on which specifically purposeful unity in nursing is established. This entails cognitive-and-affective level acceptance of the need for unity combined with the desire and the will to achieve it.

Clinical specialization in nursing is now well established, as is necessary in the light of increasing knowledge about and resulting complexity of care, and maturation in the profession. Concomitantly, some separation between specialists and generalists occurs, partly because the specialties require group association with peers to keep sharp the leading edges of the specialties and to meet a natural need for strong linkages among colleagues who hold major common interests.

Nursing is also divided in the same way and for the same reasons in accordance with areas and loci of practice or responsibility, which represents other kind of specialization. This is illustrated in public health, occupational health, and operating room nursing, and nursing administration.

Nursing is also divided, perhaps more subtly, in accordance with educational backgrounds—diploma and associate, baccalaureate, masters, or higher degree preparation. Licensed practical or vocational nurses, while recognized as essential to the provision of care in many settings, may be set apart in unnecessary ways that limit use of combined professional and practical (vocational) nursing talent on behalf of patients.

Nursing audit workshops have at one time or another included nurses in all the categories mentioned. Seeing these nurses work together in what they said was an unprecedented manner on the common goal of orientation to the audit is food for thought. There is no doubt that the pooling of talents enriched the workshops and resulted in a unity of focus on patients and their care.

Another kind of separateness is apparent, if not real distance between nursing education and nursing service. The supposedly "ivory" tower and "real" world reflect conflicting concepts; the conflict impoverishes education and service alike, as illustrated in a recent nursing journal editorial about the "two worlds of nursing."[9]

At the level of the National League for Nursing and the American Nurses' Association there is a separateness that can be related to difference in the respective national missions. On occasion, some competition between the organizations as to who should be responsible for doing what has been apparent. This is perhaps a phenomenon to be expected; both organizations are deeply committed to carrying out the responsibilities inherent in or ascribable to the missions.

In view of the disunity, some of which may be useful and some dysfunctional, it is appropriate to stress the obvious: the profession of nursing, as a whole, is responsible to society for maximum impact on the basic problem of providing personalized health care of high quality that is adequate in quantity and providing it at the lowest cost compatible with quality. Such an impact cannot be made unless there is unity in nursing in work for self-regulation in practice, including quality assurance efforts. Disunity and cross-purposes in such work might be construed in nursing, by other professionals and the public, as default in social responsibility. Pragmatically, of course, there is so much to be done in appraising and enhancing the quality of care, that it is wasteful to debate who shall do what, and productive to ask what needs to be done and who can best do it–and get it done.

As has been said, quantity, quality, and costs of care are reciprocals. Quantity of care is contingent on the number of nurses, their educational preparation, and their continuing education. Costs of care include the costs of nursing service; the economic and general welfare of nurses is essential to the provision and retention of practitioners and necessarily contributes to the costs of care. The point is that efforts pertinent to the quantity and costs of care, as well as efforts pertinent to quality, must be moral actions; the ethical base for the actions must be explicit.

To paraphrase Donabedian, values that underlie ethics in a relatively stable profession, such as nursing, tend to be largely implicit, and their influence on behavior may escape notice unless attention is directed to it. Even when decisions appear to be largely administrative or technical or political, value preferences may have been critical though concealed. As individuals, and as a profession, we must understand our own value positions and reflect them consistently in our conduct.[10] The organization of values in a value complex (ethics) which comes to characterize behavior has been seen as consistent with the development of conscience.[11] Self-regulation in nursing practice including work in quality appraisal is, above all else, a matter of conscience.

# OMEGA

We are all learning.

## References

1. Morse EV, Gordon G, Moch M: Hospital costs and quality of care: an organizational perspective. The Milbank Memorial Fund Quarterly 52(3):317, Summer 1974
2. Donabedian A: Models for organizing the delivery of personal health services and criteria for evaluating them. The Milbank Memorial Fund Quarterly 1:4, Part 2:103, 119–21, October 1972
3. Altman LK: Malpractice rates drive up doctor fees. The New York Times, July 27, 1975, pp 1, 6
4. Secretary's Commission on Malpractice. Medical Malpractice: Report of the Secretary's Commission on Medical Malpractice. Department of Health, Education and Welfare, 1973, p 60–61, 70, Washington, D.C., Superintendent of Documents, U.S. Government Printing Office Publication No. 1700 00 114
5. Hess JW: Four Years of Swimming Against the Tide: The 4-Center Experience at Detroit General Hospital, 1970-1974. Detroit, Wayne State University School of Medicine, 1974, pp 27–37

6. Danielson R: Consumer attitudes to delivery of health services. Michigan's Health, Spring 1973, p 1
7. Andropoulos S (ed): Medical cure and medical care. The Milbank Memorial Fund Quarterly 1:4, Part 2:233, October 1972
8. Lindeman CA: Research for nursing. Journal of Nursing Administration 5(6):21, July-August 1975
9. Lewis EP (ed): The two worlds of nursing. Nurs Outlook 23(7):Editorial, July 1975
10. Donabedian A: Aspects of Medical Care Administration. Cambridge, Massachusetts, Harvard University Press, 1973, pp 1, 2
11. Krathwohl DR, Bloom BS, Masia BB: Taxonomy of Educational Objectives: Handbook II, Affective Domain. New York, David McKay, 1964, pp 39, 44

# INDEX

Public health agency *(cont.)*
  statistical summary form, 84

Quality assurance, 148, 173, 178–79
  and consumer participation, 176–77
  programs, 12, 157
  research potentials related to, 177–79
  system, 12, 123–24
Quality Patient Care Scale (Qualpacs), 33, 145–46, 148–49, 151–53
Quality profile, 95–97
  regional, 175–76
  at University Hospital, 132–35
Quality review, 15, 16, 163
  and utilization review, 13
Qualpacs. *See* Quality Patient Care Scale

Random numbers, and sample selection, 185–88
Referral systems, 122
Registration, 20
Rehabilitation, 68, 88, 195
Relationship
  working, between audit committee and director of nursing service, 93, 95, 97–100
  physician-nurse, 77, 98, 99
Reliability, interrater, 72–73
Reporting and recording, 65–66, 193–94
  and continuity of care, 66, 194
  and evaluation of reported facts, 66, 193
  and minimum information, 65, 193
  to physician, 66, 193–94
Review, health care, 156–60, 162–63, 167
  functions of nurse in, 160, 162
Riehl, J.P., 100
Rosenfeld, L.S., 49
Rourke, A.J., 32
Roy, C., 100

Sample selection, directions for, 185, 188
Screening criteria, 167
Scoring instructions, for audit, 197–98
Self-regulation, in nursing, 5, 6–7, 9, 14, 15, 16, 157, 173, 177, 180, 182
Shapiro, S., 22
Shetland, M.L., 27
Siegel, H., 156
Slater Nursing Competencies Rating Scale, 33, 145–47, 151
Social Security Amendments of 1972, 12
Standards, in health care review, 161, 162
Starfield, B., 155, 156
Subjectivity, 57–58
Supervision
  of patient, 63–65, 191–92
    and nursing care plans, 64, 192
    and nursing diagnosis, 63, 191
    and patient assessment, 64, 192
  of those participating in care (except physician), 65, 192–93
    and capacity to learn, consideration of, 65, 193
    continuity and support, 65, 193
Symptoms and reactions
  and attention to patient attitude, 63, 191
  observation of, 62–63, 190–91
  related to course of disease, 62, 190–91
  and vital signs, 62–63, 191

U.S. Department of Health, Education and Welfare, 61, 191
University Hospital, University of Michigan, 125
  audit experience at, 125–38
  quality profile, 132–35
Utilization review (UR), 12–13, 15, 16, 157–58, 160
  and continuation care planning, 123

# APPENDIX 1:
# DIRECTIONS FOR SAMPLE SELECTION

## USING THE TABLE OF RANDOM NUMBERS

1. Do not use institutional or agency case record numbers for selection of cases to be audited.
2. The charts of patients discharged during the period for which the audit is to be done are numbered in sequence, from 01, 001, or 0001, up to and including the number representing the total number of charts for that period. If the total number of charts is less than 100, begin the numbering with 01; if there are more than 100 charts, begin with 001; if there are more than 1,000 charts, begin with 0001.

   The charts may be numbered on a discharge patient listing, or on discharge cards. The name of the patient and the institutional or agency case number, if any, should be indicated on the list or cards. The complete date of discharge should also be indicated on the list or cards.
3. Two or more adjacent columns from the table of random numbers should be used, as indicated by the total number of charts for discharged patients.
4. The search for identifying numbers from these columns may be made up, down, or horizontally.
5. The first number encountered in the table that matches the number on one of the charts will identify a chart to be selected for audit.
6. The search continues in the chosen direction along the columns until a second number representing a chart number is found.
7. The process is continued until the charts to be audited have been selected, in accordance with the predetermined size of the sample of charts to be audited.
8. Should the same number be encountered more than once during search of the table, it is passed over after first use of that number, and the search continues until the required number of different charts have been selected.

   The decisions needed prior to use of the selection procedure are:

   A. Choice of adjacent columns to attain the required number of digits, that is, choice of columns immediately to the left or right of the entering column

   B. Direction of search—up, down or horizontal

## Excerpt from Table of Random Numbers*

| | 00-04 | 05-09 | 10-14 | 15-19 | 20-24 | 25-29 | 30-34 | 35-39 | 40-44 | 45-49 |
|---|---|---|---|---|---|---|---|---|---|---|
| 50 | 64249 | 63664 | 39652 | 40646 | 97306 | 31741 | 07294 | 84149 | 46797 | 82487 |
| 51 | 26538 | 44249 | 04050 | 48174 | 65570 | 44072 | 40192 | 51153 | 11397 | 58212 |
| 52 | 05845 | 00512 | 78630 | 55328 | 18116 | 69296 | 91705 | 86224 | 29503 | 57071 |
| 53 | 74897 | 68373 | 67359 | 51014 | 33510 | 83048 | 17056 | 72506 | 82949 | 54600 |
| 54 | 20872 | 54570 | 35017 | 88132 | 25730 | 22626 | 86723 | 91691 | 13191 | 77212 |
| | | | | | | | | | | |
| 55 | 31432 | 96156 | 89177 | 75541 | 81355 | 24480 | 77243 | 76690 | 42507 | 84362 |
| 56 | 66890 | 61505 | 01240 | 00660 | 05873 | 13568 | 76082 | 79172 | 57913 | 93448 |
| 57 | 48194 | 57790 | 79970 | 33106 | 86904 | 48119 | 52503 | 24130 | 72824 | 21627 |
| 58 | 11303 | 87118 | 81471 | 52936 | 08555 | 28420 | 49416 | 44448 | 04269 | 27029 |
| 59 | 54374 | 57325 | 16947 | 45356 | 78371 | 10563 | 97191 | 53798 | 12693 | 27928 |
| | | | | | | | | | | |
| 60 | 64852 | 34421 | 61046 | 90849 | 13966 | 39810 | 42699 | 21753 | 76192 | 10508 |
| 61 | 16309 | 20384 | 09491 | 91588 | 97720 | 89846 | 30376 | 76970 | 23063 | 35894 |
| 62 | 42587 | 37065 | 24526 | 72602 | 57589 | 98131 | 37292 | 05967 | 26002 | 51945 |
| 63 | 40177 | 98590 | 97161 | 41682 | 84533 | 67588 | 62036 | 49967 | 01990 | 72308 |
| 64 | 82309 | 76128 | 93965 | 26743 | 24141 | 04838 | 40254 | 26065 | 07938 | 76236 |
| | | | | | | | | | | |
| 65 | 79788 | 68243 | 59732 | 04257 | 27084 | 14743 | 17520 | 95401 | 55811 | 76099 |
| 66 | 40538 | 79000 | 89559 | 25026 | 42274 | 23489 | 34502 | 75508 | 06059 | 86682 |
| 67 | 64016 | 73598 | 18609 | 73150 | 62463 | 33102 | 45205 | 87440 | 96767 | 67042 |
| 68 | 49767 | 12691 | 17903 | 93871 | 99721 | 79109 | 09425 | 29604 | 07419 | 76013 |
| 69 | 76974 | 55108 | 29795 | 08404 | 82684 | 00497 | 51126 | 79935 | 57450 | 55671 |
| | | | | | | | | | | |
| 70 | 23854 | 08480 | 85983 | 96025 | 50117 | 64610 | 99425 | 62291 | 86943 | 21541 |
| 71 | 68973 | 70551 | 25098 | 78033 | 98573 | 79848 | 31778 | 29555 | 61446 | 23037 |
| 72 | 36444 | 93600 | 65350 | 14971 | 25325 | 00427 | 52073 | 64280 | 18847 | 24768 |
| 73 | 03003 | 87800 | 07391 | 11594 | 21196 | 00781 | 32550 | 57158 | 58887 | 73041 |
| 74 | 17540 | 26188 | 36647 | 78386 | 04558 | 61463 | 57842 | 90382 | 77019 | 24210 |
| | | | | | | | | | | |
| 75 | 38916 | 55809 | 47982 | 41968 | 69760 | 79422 | 80154 | 91486 | 19180 | 15100 |
| 76 | 64288 | 19843 | 69122 | 42502 | 48508 | 28820 | 59933 | 72998 | 99942 | 10515 |
| 77 | 86809 | 51564 | 38040 | 39418 | 49915 | 19000 | 58050 | 16899 | 79952 | 57849 |
| 78 | 99800 | 99566 | 14742 | 05028 | 30033 | 94889 | 53381 | 23656 | 75787 | 59223 |
| 79 | 92345 | 31890 | 95712 | 08279 | 91794 | 94068 | 49337 | 88674 | 35355 | 12267 |
| | | | | | | | | | | |
| 80 | 90363 | 65162 | 32245 | 82279 | 79256 | 80834 | 06088 | 99462 | 56705 | 06118 |
| 81 | 64437 | 32242 | 48431 | 04835 | 39070 | 59702 | 31508 | 60935 | 22390 | 52246 |
| 82 | 91714 | 53662 | 28373 | 34333 | 55791 | 74758 | 51144 | 18827 | 10704 | 76803 |
| 83 | 20902 | 17646 | 31391 | 31459 | 33315 | 03444 | 55743 | 74701 | 58851 | 27427 |
| 84 | 12217 | 86007 | 70371 | 52281 | 14510 | 76094 | 96579 | 54853 | 78339 | 20839 |
| | | | | | | | | | | |
| 85 | 45177 | 02863 | 42307 | 53571 | 22532 | 74921 | 17735 | 42201 | 80540 | 54721 |
| 86 | 28325 | 90814 | 08804 | 52746 | 47913 | 54577 | 47525 | 77705 | 95330 | 21866 |
| 87 | 29019 | 28776 | 56116 | 54791 | 64604 | 08815 | 46049 | 71186 | 34650 | 14994 |
| 88 | 84979 | 81353 | 56219 | 67062 | 26146 | 82567 | 33122 | 14124 | 46240 | 92973 |
| 89 | 50371 | 26347 | 48513 | 63915 | 11158 | 25563 | 91915 | 18431 | 92978 | 11591 |

| | 00-04 | 05-09 | 10-14 | 15-19 | 20-24 | 25-29 | 30-34 | 35-39 | 40-44 | 45-49 |
|---|---|---|---|---|---|---|---|---|---|---|
| 90 | 53422 | 06825 | 69711 | 67950 | 64716 | 18003 | 49581 | 45378 | 99878 | 61130 |
| 91 | 67453 | 35651 | 89316 | 41620 | 32048 | 70225 | 47597 | 33137 | 31443 | 51445 |
| 92 | 07294 | 85353 | 74819 | 23445 | 68237 | 07202 | 99515 | 62282 | 53809 | 26685 |
| 93 | 79544 | 00302 | 45338 | 16015 | 66613 | 88968 | 14595 | 63836 | 77716 | 79596 |
| 94 | 64144 | 85442 | 82060 | 46471 | 24162 | 39500 | 87351 | 36637 | 42833 | 71875 |
| | | | | | | | | | | |
| 95 | 90919 | 11883 | 58318 | 00042 | 52402 | 28210 | 34075 | 33272 | 00840 | 73268 |
| 96 | 06670 | 57353 | 86275 | 92276 | 77591 | 46924 | 60839 | 55437 | 03183 | 13191 |
| 97 | 36634 | 93976 | 52062 | 83678 | 41256 | 60948 | 18685 | 48992 | 19462 | 96062 |
| 98 | 75101 | 72891 | 85745 | 67106 | 26010 | 62107 | 60885 | 37503 | 55461 | 71213 |
| 99 | 05112 | 71222 | 72654 | 51583 | 05228 | 62056 | 57390 | 42746 | 39272 | 96659 |

| | 50-54 | 55-59 | 60-64 | 65-69 | 70-74 | 75-79 | 80-84 | 85-89 | 90-94 | 95-99 |
|---|---|---|---|---|---|---|---|---|---|---|
| 50 | 32847 | 31282 | 03345 | 89593 | 69214 | 70381 | 78285 | 20054 | 91018 | 16742 |
| 51 | 16916 | 00041 | 30236 | 55023 | 14253 | 76582 | 12092 | 86533 | 92426 | 37655 |
| 52 | 66176 | 34047 | 21005 | 27137 | 03191 | 48970 | 64625 | 22394 | 39622 | 79085 |
| 53 | 46299 | 13335 | 12180 | 16861 | 38043 | 59292 | 62675 | 63631 | 37020 | 78195 |
| 54 | 22847 | 47839 | 45385 | 23289 | 47526 | 54098 | 45683 | 55849 | 51575 | 64689 |
| | | | | | | | | | | |
| 55 | 41851 | 54160 | 92320 | 69936 | 34803 | 92479 | 33399 | 71160 | 74777 | 83378 |
| 56 | 28444 | 59497 | 91586 | 95917 | 68553 | 28639 | 06455 | 34174 | 11130 | 91994 |
| 57 | 47520 | 62378 | 98855 | 83174 | 13088 | 16561 | 68559 | 26679 | 06238 | 51254 |
| 58 | 34978 | 63271 | 13142 | 82681 | 05271 | 08822 | 06490 | 44984 | 49307 | 62717 |
| 59 | 37404 | 80416 | 69035 | 92980 | 49486 | 74378 | 75610 | 74976 | 70056 | 15478 |
| | | | | | | | | | | |
| 60 | 32400 | 65482 | 52099 | 53676 | 74648 | 94148 | 65095 | 69597 | 52771 | 71551 |
| 61 | 89262 | 86332 | 51718 | 70663 | 11623 | 29834 | 79820 | 73002 | 84886 | 03591 |
| 62 | 86866 | 09127 | 98021 | 03871 | 27789 | 58444 | 44832 | 36505 | 40672 | 30180 |
| 63 | 90814 | 14833 | 08759 | 74645 | 05046 | 94056 | 99094 | 65091 | 32663 | 73040 |
| 64 | 19192 | 82756 | 20553 | 58446 | 55376 | 88914 | 75096 | 26119 | 83898 | 43816 |
| | | | | | | | | | | |
| 65 | 77585 | 52593 | 56612 | 95766 | 10019 | 29531 | 73064 | 20953 | 53523 | 58136 |
| 66 | 23757 | 16364 | 05096 | 03192 | 62386 | 45389 | 85332 | 18877 | 55710 | 96459 |
| 67 | 45989 | 96257 | 23850 | 26216 | 23309 | 21526 | 07425 | 50254 | 19455 | 29315 |
| 68 | 92970 | 94243 | 07316 | 41467 | 64837 | 52406 | 25225 | 51553 | 31220 | 14032 |
| 69 | 74346 | 59596 | 40088 | 98176 | 17896 | 86900 | 20249 | 77753 | 19099 | 48885 |
| | | | | | | | | | | |
| 70 | 87646 | 41309 | 27636 | 45153 | 29988 | 94770 | 07255 | 70908 | 05340 | 99751 |
| 71 | 50099 | 71038 | 45146 | 06146 | 55211 | 99429 | 43169 | 66259 | 97786 | 59180 |
| 72 | 10127 | 46900 | 64984 | 75348 | 04115 | 33624 | 68774 | 60013 | 35515 | 62556 |
| 73 | 67995 | 81977 | 18984 | 64091 | 02785 | 27762 | 42529 | 97144 | 80407 | 64524 |
| 74 | 26304 | 80217 | 84934 | 82657 | 69291 | 35397 | 98714 | 35104 | 08187 | 48109 |
| | | | | | | | | | | |
| 75 | 81994 | 41070 | 56642 | 64091 | 31229 | 02595 | 13513 | 45148 | 78722 | 30144 |
| 76 | 59537 | 34662 | 79631 | 89403 | 65212 | 09975 | 06118 | 86197 | 58208 | 16162 |
| 77 | 51228 | 10937 | 62396 | 81460 | 47331 | 91403 | 95007 | 06047 | 16846 | 64809 |
| 78 | 31089 | 37995 | 29577 | 07828 | 42272 | 54016 | 21950 | 86192 | 99046 | 84864 |
| 79 | 38207 | 97938 | 93459 | 75174 | 79460 | 55436 | 57206 | 87644 | 21296 | 43395 |

|    | 50-54 | 55-59 | 60-64 | 65-69 | 70-74 | 75-79 | 80-84 | 85-89 | 90-94 | 95-99 |
|----|-------|-------|-------|-------|-------|-------|-------|-------|-------|-------|
| 80 | 88666 | 31142 | 09474 | 89712 | 63153 | 62333 | 42212 | 06140 | 42594 | 43671 |
| 81 | 53365 | 56134 | 67582 | 92557 | 89520 | 33452 | 05134 | 70628 | 27612 | 33738 |
| 82 | 89807 | 74530 | 38004 | 91202 | 11693 | 90257 | 05500 | 79920 | 62700 | 43325 |
| 83 | 18682 | 81038 | 85662 | 90915 | 91631 | 22223 | 91588 | 80774 | 07716 | 12548 |
| 84 | 63571 | 32579 | 63942 | 25371 | 09234 | 94592 | 98475 | 76884 | 37635 | 33608 |
| 85 | 68927 | 56492 | 67799 | 95398 | 77642 | 54913 | 91853 | 08424 | 81450 | 76229 |
| 86 | 56401 | 63186 | 39389 | 88798 | 31356 | 89235 | 97036 | 32341 | 33292 | 73757 |
| 87 | 24333 | 95603 | 02359 | 72942 | 46287 | 95382 | 08452 | 62862 | 97869 | 71775 |
| 88 | 17025 | 84202 | 95199 | 62272 | 06366 | 16175 | 97577 | 99304 | 41587 | 03686 |
| 89 | 02804 | 08253 | 52133 | 20224 | 68034 | 50865 | 57868 | 22343 | 55111 | 03607 |
| 90 | 08298 | 03879 | 20995 | 19850 | 73090 | 13191 | 18963 | 82244 | 78479 | 99121 |
| 91 | 59883 | 01785 | 82403 | 96062 | 03785 | 03488 | 12970 | 64896 | 38336 | 30030 |
| 92 | 46982 | 06682 | 62864 | 91837 | 74021 | 89094 | 39952 | 64158 | 79614 | 78235 |
| 93 | 31121 | 47266 | 07661 | 02051 | 67599 | 24471 | 69843 | 83696 | 74102 | 76287 |
| 94 | 97867 | 56641 | 63416 | 17577 | 30161 | 87320 | 37752 | 73276 | 48969 | 41915 |
| 95 | 37364 | 86746 | 08415 | 14621 | 49430 | 23311 | 15836 | 72492 | 49372 | 44103 |
| 96 | 09559 | 26263 | 69511 | 28064 | 75999 | 44540 | 13337 | 10918 | 79846 | 54809 |
| 97 | 53873 | 55571 | 00608 | 42661 | 91332 | 63956 | 74087 | 59008 | 47493 | 99581 |
| 98 | 35531 | 19162 | 86406 | 05299 | 77511 | 24311 | 57257 | 22826 | 77555 | 05941 |
| 99 | 28229 | 88629 | 26595 | 94932 | 30721 | 16197 | 78742 | 34974 | 97528 | 45447 |

C. Category of columns to which the search will move; for example, to successive 5's, 10's, and so forth

D. Location of columns at top or bottom of page should additional numbers be needed for identifying the desired total of cases required for the sample

At one time or another, there may be a wish to develop a randomized sample of charts for patients in special clinical or other categories. In this event, stratified random selection is advised, and the reader is referred to Snedecor's text on *Statistical Methods* for details of the process.

# APPENDIX 2:
# EXPLANATION OF AUDIT SCHEDULE COMPONENTS

## FUNCTIONS AND SUBCOMPONENTS

### Function I. Application and Execution of Physician's Legal Orders

1. *Medical Diagnosis Complete.* The diagnosis is clear enough to permit intelligent execution of the nursing functions. A diagnosis which conforms in terminology with that of the International Classification of Diseases, published by the U.S. Department of Health, Education and Welfare, ordinarily suffices.

    At varying points in patient care, as when clinically unexplained changes occur, the maximum nursing base may be a tentative clinical diagnosis or other significant data that justify intervention.

    Where patients have multiple diagnoses, the same rules apply. Here, one of the hazards in nursing and for the patient, however, is that the primary diagnosis in relation to which care is being given remains the sole focus of care, whereas the other diseases or disorders involved may be equally important in the nursing process. The patient who had cholecystitis with cholecystectomy, and also has longstanding diabetes mellitus, may receive much nursing attention for the surgical problem but only cursory attention to his problems with diabetes.

2. *Orders Complete.* The physician's orders are clear, explicit, and conclusive *when looked at in regard to the patient, as well as to the diagnosis and other clinical data.* Orders for medications should include the dosage and frequency of administration, and the route of administration (unless it is clear from the nature of the medication, as for aspirin or insulin). Orders should be specific not only when medications are administered by the

**195**

nurse, but also when self-administered by the patient or given by family members or other responsible persons.
3. *Orders Current.* Orders are up to date according to pertinent institutional or agency policy *and* nursing judgment. For example, an order for Seconal may fall within the stop-order policy limit. But if there is evidence that Seconal is causing untoward effects in the patient, the nurse will withhold the medication and consult the physician about the situation rather than adhere to policy only.
4. *Orders Promptly Executed.* The chart shows reasonable and appropriate timing between the giving of the order and compliance with it. There should be adherence to institutional or agency policy in regard to the dating of the orders, the recording of the time at which the orders are written, and the recording of the date and time of execution of the orders.
5. *Evidence That the Nurse Understood Cause and Effect.* The chart shows that the nurse knew what she was doing and why she was doing it. A nurse performing any service ordered by the physician is legally obligated to understand the cause and effect of that service before performing it. The nurse is required to understand not only the basis for and anticipated therapeutic results of performance, but also the possible side effects of other complications. It cannot be too strongly emphasized that the nurse's right to perform any function is absolutely contingent upon her ability to understand its underlying reason and its anticipated effect, as well as upon her ability to perform the function.
6. *Evidence That the Nurse Took the Health History Into Account.* The chart reflects recognition that knowledge of pertinent points in the patient's past pattern of health and illness are vital to intelligent current nursing care. The purpose of the history is to develop data from which to make nursing assessments of strengths, weaknesses, and life style which are taken into account when planning nursing intervention relative to health-illness problems.

## Function II. Observations of Symptoms and Reactions

7. *Related to the Course of the Above Disease in General.* There is evidence that the nurse understands the disease in the textbook or classic sense and is observing the patient with the classic picture as her clinical frame of reference.
   By this is meant that the natural history of the disease from which the patient suffers should be known by the nurse and used as the clinical base for developing the nursing process. In this regard, the paradigm developed by Leavell and Clark is useful because it depicts the pattern of movement through prepathogenesis, early pathogenesis, discernible early disease, advanced disease, and convalescence, with possible outcomes of recovery, a chronic state, disability, or death.
8. *Related to the Course of the Above Disease in This Patient.* There is evidence that, in addition to the knowledge of the disease in item 7, there are observations of the patient's individual response to the disease and its treatment.
   This simply means progression from consideration of the natural history of the disease in any man and the natural history of the disease in the par-

ticular man, which may be influenced by his heredity, his general health, and his life situation, as well as by his treatment and response to treatment.

9. *Related Complications Due to Therapy (Each Medication and Each Treatment).* Recorded observations relate to expected therapeutic and possible or unexpected untoward side effects.

    The observations are one reflection of the nurse's ability to understand cause and effect relationships in nursing management.

10. *Vital Signs.* When indicated by the patient's situation, recording includes: temperature; quality of pulse, as well as rhythm and rate; quality of respirations, as well as rate; blood pressure; tone, temperature, and color of the skin; and observations pertinent to feeling tone—that is, the patient's affective state.

    Here the emphasis is on collection of data so that patterns and trends in the vital signs are clear. The recording of a single vital sign, such as one blood pressure determination, is meaningless because it is the trend in blood pressures that indicates need for, and response to, therapy.

11. *Patient to His Condition.* There is evidence that attention was given to the patient's attitude toward his clinical condition and life situation as it influences and is influenced by the clinical condition.

    "Attention" means careful consideration of behaviors reflective of attitude. This includes use of direct, indirect, and reflective questions to the patient aimed at eliciting attitudinal responses, as well as observation of nonverbal behavior.

12. *Patient to His Course of Disease.* There is evidence that attention was given to the demonstrable degree of the patient's understanding and acceptance, rejection, or ambivalence toward his specific disease and illness.

    Attention here is literally twofold: attention to the disease that is to the pathological process; and attention to the illness that is the acute or chronic manifestations of the pathologic process. For example, it is possible for a patient to reject his disease but to accept the illness it causes, or to accept the disease but reject his illness. Nursing intervention carried out without recognition of the patient's position will fall short of its mark.

## Function III. Supervision of the Patient

13. *Evidence That Initial Nursing Diagnosis Was Made.* The chart shows that nursing problems were determined and categorized as the basis for nursing care plans directed toward solution of the problems. This diagnosis should be made as soon as possible after the first nursing contact with the patient. In some charts, nursing care plans strongly suggest that a diagnosis was made. In this event, evidence of the implicit diagnosis should be taken into account.

    Since "to determine" means to establish after consideration, investigation, or calculation, and "to categorize" means to classify into specified divisions, it is obvious that initial "nursing diagnosis" as here used encompasses the steps in the nursing process up to the point of formulation of the plan of care.

14. *Safety of the Patient.* There is recorded evidence of precautions taken to prevent physical injury.

These precautions include assistance in early ambulation and other activities involving neuromuscular functions which are difficult for the patient and encompass environmental safeguards as well.

15. *Security of the Patient.* There is evidence of work that helps in maintaining a therapeutic environment for the patient.

This work includes support of productive interpersonal relationships, as well as attention to the physical setting in which the human interactions occur.

16. *Adaptation (Support of Patient in Reactions to Condition and Care).* There is evidence of attempts to help the patient adjust to his changing condition, to the course of his illness, to his care, and to his anticipated future.

These attempts include helping the patient to accept attainable therapeutic goals; helping reduce the patient's anxiety, fear, and doubt; helping him toward self-confidence and confidence in his care; and helping the patient to exert the physical and emotional efforts required in his situation, in accordance with his capacities.

17. *Continuing Assessment of Patient's Condition and Capacity.* The chart reflects ongoing evaluation of the current status and situation of the patient and the effects of care, with analysis of current nursing problems.

This continuing assessment involves both the collection of data with validation of them and interpretation of that data with validation of the interpretation as a base for modification or revision of the plan of care.

18. *Nursing Care Plans Changed in Accordance with Assessment.* There is evidence that the plan of care was adapted as nursing problems were altered by changes in the patient's condition and capacity.

In relation to assessment, the difference between this and item 17 is that item 17 emphasized continuity of assessment, as opposed to assessment of one or another single aspect of the patient's condition or capacity.

This subcomponent, however, is primarily addressed to the question of whether the nursing care plan was appropriately altered as the patient's condition and capacity changed.

19. *Interaction with the Family and with Other People Considered.* There is evidence of concern for the people in contact with the patient, with a view toward promoting interactions that are beneficial to all concerned.

This means that the patient's interactions with his family, his physician, and other people important to them are observed with respect to the interests and concerns reflected therein by them, and use of those observations to advance mutually constructive relationships.

## Function IV. Supervision of Those Participating in Care (Except the Physician)

20. *Care Taught to Patient, Family, or Others Participating in His Care.* The chart reflects what care was taught, what guidance and support were given, to whom, and by whom accomplished.

The care taught includes all activities resumed or assumed by the patient and all the tasks performed by others involved in his care. It is assumed that care has not been taught until the behavior of those taught shows or suggests that learning has occurred.

21. *Physical, Mental, and Emotional Capacity to Learn Considered.* The evidence shows that the ability and readiness of those to be taught, guided, and supported were taken into account.
    Consideration of the learner's capacity includes initial and continuing assessments of the need for and the appropriateness of that which is to be taught, in relation to the ability and the readiness of those being taught.
22. *Continuity of Supervision to Those Taught.* The evidence shows that the results of initial and additional teaching were assessed with appropriate follow-up.
    This subcomponent is also based on the assumption of item 20 that teaching has not occurred until it is reflected in the behavior of the learners, and that activities and tasks in self-care or care given by others are not ordinarily learned through a single exposure to "teaching." The emphasis here is on the follow-up.
23. *Support of Those Giving Care.* The chart reflects the giving of emotional and physical help to those taught and supervised.
    Here the emphasis is on continuing assessment of the ability and readiness of those taught, with appropriate action in accordance with the assessment.

## Function V. Reporting and Recording

24. *Facts on Which Further Care Depended Were Recorded.* The information recorded facilitated continuing physician and nurse management of clinical care.
    Minimum information includes observations of symptoms and reactions; evidence of the execution of physician's orders; and data developed as part of the supervision of the patient.
25. *Essential Facts Reported to the Physician.* The chart shows that basic necessary information was conveyed to the physician either in writing or verbally. The facts may be major or minor; it is their importance to the physician and his management of the patient's care that makes them essential or nonessential.
    Essential facts are those indispensable to patient-centered care, as well as those that are clinically significant as discrete facts.
26. *Reporting of Facts Included Evaluation Thereof.* There is evidence that, in reporting facts, nursing judgment concerning their significance or possible importance is included.
    In other words, the emphasis here is on nursing expression of the reason why the facts were considered indispensable to the physician in the management of his patient.
27. *Patient and Family Alerted as to What to Report to the Physician.* There is evidence that patient or family members are directed to report to the physician those factors, signs, symptoms, or situations the direct reporting of which is conducive to patient and family rapport with the physician, or is otherwise mutually advantageous.
    The intent here is to foster communications with the physician about questions which the nurse cannot properly answer, or questions the answering of which by the physician serves a special purpose in the management of

medical or nursing care. One special purpose would be to have anxieties and fears allayed by the physician when he can best accomplish this.

Having the patient and family members report to the physician does not relieve the nurse of responsibility for direct reporting to the physician. In critical matters, the physician may be assisted by receiving separate communications from the patient or family and from the nurse.

28. *The Chart Permitted Continuity of Care.* The chart permits an uninterrupted sequence of care from nurse to nurse, from nurse to physician, and from nurse to other professionals. It is of major importance that the chart indicate succinctly that information vital to the patient's therapeutic regimen was reported to the physician.

The question to be answered in this subcomponent is not whether there actually was continuity in care, but whether continuity of care was possible with use of the information on the chart.

## Function VI. Application and Execution of Nursing Procedures and Techniques

29. *Administration of Medications/Supervision of Their Use.* Whether medications are given by the nurse, or whether the nurse is supervising the patient or the family in the taking or giving, the chart reflects nurse or patient and family awareness of expected therapeutic results and possible untoward side effects.

For every medication, including those administered by the physician, there are anticipated therapeutic effects and possible untoward side effects, including reactions of intolerance and idiosyncrasy. Wherever more than one medication is used, the possibility of drug incompatibility must also be considered.

30. *Personal Care (Bathing, Oral Hygiene, Skin, Nail, and Hair Care).* The chart indicates appropriate attention to personal care whether the care activities are performed by the patient, a family member, or another person.

Appropriate attention includes not only concern with cleanliness, but also with grooming conducive to feelings of well-being, personal worth, and dignity.

31. *Nutrition, Including Special Diets.* There is evidence of attention to adequate nutrition as appropriate to the patient's condition, course, and stage of growth and development. If a special diet is used, there is evidence as to whether or not, and to what extent, the diet and the main reasons for it appear to be understood and accepted by the patient and his family.

Appraisal of the patient's usual eating habits is a part of nursing assessment, whether the patient is on a regular or a special diet. Results are used in formulating and implementing nursing care plans.

32. *Fluid and Electrolyte Balance.* The chart reflects consideration of possible disturbances in body fluid and electrolyte balance, as indicated by the patient's age, condition, and course of illness.

Considerations of possible disturbances include attention to fluid intake and urinary output; changes in respiratory rate and depth; changes in skin turgor; dryness of skin and mucous membranes; changes in behavior, such as increasing apathy or restlessness; thirst; ascites; and edema.

33. *Elimination.* Evidence that bowel function is considered, and that appro-

priate action is taken when the patient's bowels are not functioning normally for him.

The emphasis should be on what is normal for the patient in health and the deviations that occur because of his illness. Action should follow the patient's pattern as closely as permitted by his condition.

34. *Rest and Sleep.* Evidence that the patient's usual and unusual patterns of rest and sleep are taken into account in planning his regimen and supervising his care.

Appraisal of the patterns of rest and sleep is also a part of nursing assessment. It permits planning of the regimen with regard to rest and sleep, to follow as closely as possible the patient's natural rhythms. If the usual patterns obviously yield deficits in rest and sleep, the regimen should be planned with the aim of bringing about appropriate alterations of the pattern.

35. *Physical Activity.* The chart shows the relationship between the activity in which the patient engages and the activity which is clinically permissible. Where excess or deficit is found, efforts are made to reconcile actual physical activity with clinically estimated physical tolerance.

Development of a balance between too much and too little activity requires that the patient understand and accept the reasons that underlie restriction or increase in activity.

36. *Irrigations of Wounds, Canals, Cavities.* Evidence that irrigations are performed as ordered; the results; and, if dressings are used, what kind and whether sterile or clean.

This subcomponent refers to all types of irrigation and includes enemas. If problems in performance of the procedure arise either in relation to the irrigation or in relation to patient reaction to it, they should be recorded.

37. *Dressings and Bandages.* Evidence that these are applied as ordered or as indicated. Topical applications, if any, should be identified; the kind of dressing used and whether it was sterile or clean should be noted.

Observations of the wound site and adjacent tissues should be recorded in a manner that permits continuing appraisal of progress in healing and early detection of complications.

38. *Formal Exercise Program.* Indication that a treatment plan is carried out as ordered by the physician or as outlined by a physical therapist at the physician's request.

Here, the nurse is responsible for seeing that the program is carried on and also that supportive encouragement and assistance are given to the patient.

39. *Rehabilitation (Other Than Formal Exercises).* Evidence of teaching or encouragement toward independent living—range of motion (ROM), active and passive exercises, activities of daily living (ADL), use of aids in ADL. If nursing rehabilitation is not required, there is evidence that the nursing care approach is restorative in nature.

Activities of daily living require motivation and participation in decision making which leads to the activities, as well as to the ability to perform them. Evaluation of the performance may increase or decrease motivation. At best, encouragement from the nurse reflects knowledge and understanding of this. The restorative approach has the same foundation. Activities of daily living include not only self-care but also other activities which give a positive meaning to the day for the patient.

40. *Prevention of Complications, Including Infections.* Evidence of work toward

maintenance of hygiene, early detection of primary or secondary infections or other untoward symptoms; early detection of complications due to therapy; and prevention of avoidable disabilities, such as contractures.

Consideration of complications that might reasonably be expected, or prevented, is a part of initial and ongoing nursing assessment.

41. *Recreation and Diversion.* The chart indicates specific attention to the patient's need for activities that interest and amuse him and divert his attention from disease and illness.

For counteracting disease- and illness-oriented tasks, activities, and limitations, the importance of recreation and diversion, however simple the related activities may be, cannot be overemphasized as part of orientation toward health.

42. *Clinical Procedures.* The chart shows results of urinalyses and other examinations done by nurses, if any; blood pressure determinations; and results of performance of other general nursing procedures.

43. *Special Treatments, Including Tracheostomy Management, Use of Oxygen, Colostomy Care, Gastric Feedings, Care of Decubiti, etc.* Evidence that the treatments were performed, indication of results, and evaluation thereof; observations pertinent to patient's physical and emotional reactions.

The preparation of the patient for the special treatment is a part of the performance of special treatments. Patient's preferences as to the way in which the procedure is to be performed should be recognized and adhered to, as well as possible. Where it is not safe to follow his preference, the record should indicate efforts to explain this and to enlist his cooperation.

44. *Procedures and Techniques Taught to Patient.* Evidence that any procedure or technique the patient can learn to carry out to his advantage is in fact taught.

This subcomponent is addressed to the development of increasing independence in self-care by the patient, within the limits of feasibility for him.

## Function VII. Promotion of Physical and Emotional Health By Direction and Teaching

45. *Plans for Medical Emergency.* Evidence that, by policy or by specific teaching, patient, family, and other personnel know what to do in situations which are acutely worrisome or dangerous for the patient and which arouse anxiety or fear in those responsible for his care.

Planning for medical emergencies is contingent on assessment of the emergencies that might reasonably be expected to arise, in terms of what the patient and his family perceive as constituting an emergency and what is clinically perceived as an emergency situation.

In accredited hospitals and nursing homes, there are specific policies for the management of major emergency situations. In auditing, it is necessary to note whether policies were carried out as necessary.

In public health nursing agencies, plans about what to do if medical emergencies arise are developed with patient and family and in conjunction with the physician, if the patient is under private medical care. If the patient is not under private care, the patient and his family should know precisely what clinical facility to use in an emergency, and how to use it.

46. *Emotional Support for the Patient.* Evidence of work toward helping the patient understand and accept his feelings about himself, his condition, and his care, and helping him develop his coping abilities and other potentials.

    Provision of emotional support requires assessment of the special needs of the patient, his characteristic behaviors, and his psychosocial and cultural matrix. Without this data base, it is unlikely that the rapport and open communication necessary for providing emotional support will be achieved.

47. *Emotional Support for the Family.* The chart reflects impressions and facts about family reactions toward the patient and his condition, which can be used to help the family accept the patient's condition and their own feelings about it.

    Providing emotional support for the family requires the same data base as that required in emotional support of the patient.

48. *Teaching Preventive Health Care.* Evidence of promoting and protecting the health of the patient and his family, and of teaching about secondary prevention, that is, teaching the early detection of signs and symptoms which may indicate new disorders or complications due to established disease.

    Assessment of the goals and motivation of the patient and family precedes discussion and use of selected educational tools with them. The teaching plan will be unique for the patient and his family, and its effectiveness dependent on the rapport already established. Minimally, patient and family need to understand the medical and nursing regimen and to understand, accept, and carry out the necessary procedures and activities.

49. *Evaluation of the Need for Additional Resources, Including Spiritual Guidance, Social Services, Occupational Therapy, or Continuity of Nursing Care Under Another Aegis; Homemaker Service.* Evidence that, when indicated, possible needs for consultation or direct service were assessed.

    Evaluation of the need for use of additional resources should occur periodically throughout the time the patient is under care. Continuation care planning should be done well in advance of the patient's discharge.

50. *Action Taken in Regard to Needs Identified.* Evidence that nursing action was taken, with the knowledge of the patient's attending physician, for needs identified as relating to the promotion, by direction and teaching, of the patient's physical and emotional health.

    It is of course useless to identify and categorize needs and problems unless action is taken directly or indirectly to help meet the needs and to solve or alleviate the problems.

# SCORING INSTRUCTIONS

The auditor will have checked (√) the box of her choice for each of the 50 subcomponents in Part II of the audit schedule.

1. Establish the score for each of the functions by adding the sum of the checked items in each column. Enter this number in the indicated box.
2. Add the scores for the seven functions to obtain the total score. Enter this number in the indicated box.

## "Does Not Apply" Values Guide

| Total of "Does Not Apply" Items | "Does Not Apply" Score Value |
|:---:|:---:|
| 0 | 1.00 |
| 2 | 1.01 |
| 3 or 4 | 1.02 |
| 5 or 6 | 1.03 |
| 7 or 8 | 1.04 |
| 9 or 10 | 1.05 |
| 11 or 12 | 1.06 |
| 13 or 14 | 1.07 |
| 15 | 1.08 |
| 16 or 17 | 1.09 |
| 18 or 19 | 1.10 |
| 20 | 1.11 |
| 21 or 22 | 1.12 |
| 23 | 1.13 |
| 24 or 25 | 1.14 |
| 26 | 1.15 |
| 27 or 28 | 1.16 |
| 29 | 1.17 |
| 30 or 31 | 1.18 |
| 32 | 1.19 |
| 33 or 34 | 1.20 |
| 35 | 1.21 |
| 36 | 1.22 |
| 37 or 38 | 1.23 |
| 39 | 1.24 |
| 40 | 1.25 |
| 41 | 1.26 |
| 42 or 43 | 1.27 |
| 44 | 1.28 |
| 45 | 1.29 |
| 46 | 1.30 |
| 47 | 1.31 |
| 48 or 49 | 1.32 |
| 50 | 1.33 |

3. The Does not apply column is added separately (Functions VI and VII). The score for the Does not apply items is the sum of the checked items for each of these two functions. Enter this number in indicated box.
4. Select the appropriate score value for the Does not apply score values guide below.
5. To obtain the final audit score, multiply the total score by the appropriate Does not apply score value. Enter the final score on Part III of the audit schedule.